BEING
WELL

with Chronic Illness

BEING
WELL

with Chronic Illness

A Guide to Joy & Resilience
with Your Diagnosis

KAT HILL & NANCY PEATE

Hatherleigh Press is committed to preserving
and protecting the natural resources of the earth.
Environmentally responsible and sustainable practices
are embraced within the company's mission statement.

Visit us at www.hatherleighpress.com and register online
for free offers, discounts, special events, and more.

BEING WELL WITH CHRONIC ILLNESS

Library of Congress Cataloging-in-Publication Data is available.

ISBN: 978-157826-947-1

Printed in the United States

10 9 8 7 6 5 4 3 2 1

Medical Disclaimer: No individual should use the
information in this book for self-diagnosis or to self-
treat any condition. Exercise should not be initiated
without first consulting your healthcare provider.
You are responsible for your own health and safety.

For Ken, Emma, Nastassia, and Sawyer:

My foundation, my heart, my family

—Kat

For Rob and Declan:

My guys, always

—Nancy

✳ CONTENTS

Preface		ix
Chapter 1:	**THE JOURNEY TO WELLNESS**	**1**
Chapter 2:	**THE WELLNESS SPIRAL**	**11**
Chapter 3:	**THE RABBIT HOLE**	**25**
Chapter 4:	**CROSSROADS**	**41**
Chapter 5:	**COMPASSION FOR SELF AND OTHERS**	**61**
Chapter 6:	**COMMUNITY**	**81**
Chapter 7:	**JOY AND CONTENTMENT**	**97**
Chapter 8:	**INTENTIONAL WELLNESS**	**115**
Chapter 9:	**HEALTH CARE TEAM**	**131**
Chapter 10:	**BEING WELL**	**147**
Afterword		163
Acknowledgements		165
Further Reading		167
Resources		169
Bibliography		175
About the Authors		177

✳ PREFACE

WE MET BY CHANCE soon after we were diagnosed. We come to you with full lives not defined by illness. We are a healthcare provider and a reference librarian who have nurtured successful careers and raised children. We are mothers and daughters, wives and sisters, dancers and drummers, friends and fighters. We have Parkinson's, a progressive nervous system disorder, and we are thriving.

We have learned ways to be well while living with chronic illness. We have found our village in early morning boxing bootcamps, local hospital conference rooms, and dance studios. We have looked for our people at the city, state, national, and international levels, and have found them at conferences, colleges, and congresses.

We find strength in our numbers. We enjoy new friendships. We find laughter and hope over coffee. It has been said that you will never meet a nicer group of people than those who have Parkinson's, and this has certainly been true for us. We are proud to introduce some of them to you in the following chapters.

Our boxing coach has helped us come together to fight more than a punching bag. We are fighting for our lives. What started out as a 6:30AM workout four days a week has grown into the foundation for a tight group of fighters battling this incurable brain disease.

We are easy to spot in our boxing class. Nancy's workout shirt says, "Parkinson's Picked the Wrong Girl to Mess With," and Kat has painted cheerful, purple polka dots on her boxing gloves.

Even before receiving the formal diagnosis, we sought information. We sought knowledge about symptoms we were experiencing and ways to improve our health. We learned that exercise and staying social are the only things known to slow the progression of this disease. Medicines help to treat symptoms, but there is no cure.

Parkinson's is a brain disease with an unknown cause. It is the second most common brain disease after Alzheimer's. According to the Parkinson's Foundation, more people have Parkinson's than the combined number of people with multiple sclerosis, muscular dystrophy, and amyotrophic lateral sclerosis (ALS) disease. One-third of those who are affected, are women.

We believe that by sharing information and our stories, we make it easier for those who follow. Our intention is to convey authentically our grief, hope, and compassion. Our stories include choosing joy over despair and health over illness. We illustrate our ways of navigating a diagnosis and offer a framework for shaping positive thinking about your own journey.

This book is for anyone whose life has been touched by chronic illness. Chapter by chapter, we guide you through the process of finding your natural strengths as you define your story. We will ask you in italic text to try a reflective activity. Consider having a pen or other way to make notes as you read. We also give you a glimpse into the lives of some amazing people and discuss tools that you can use to *be well*. We guide you through ways to approach your experience and show you how to embrace gratitude and positivity in your life.

We hope that this book will inspire you to choose joy in those times when you need it most.

Be well,
—Kat and Nancy

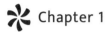 Chapter 1

THE JOURNEY TO WELLNESS

"Sometimes you have to let go of the picture of what you thought it would be like and learn to find joy in the story you are actually living."

—Rachel Marie Martin

WE ARE ALL ON a journey.

It has taken us time to recognize that we have a role and a voice in choosing the path that our journey takes, and we would like to share with you tools for how to use your mind and voice. We did not start out seeing a clear map to follow, nor did we receive a checklist of what we would need on our way. We are two women good at planning, yet somehow, we ended up on a trip without a map!

Your journey will be your own; no two are the same. However, like us, you will come to many crossroads, face many obstacles, and have many choices to make along the way. We think you are in charge of your wellness, and in charge of how you choose to think about it. Come along with us and let's get started with experiencing health in a new way.

AWAKENING

When you were young, did your dreams include having a chronic illness? Probably not! It may have never even crossed your mind. We dreamed of fairies and ballerinas. Our dreams never included a chronic illness. But now as adults, we dream big and choose to integrate our dreams with the reality of living with Parkinson's disease. Your experience may include a different diagnosis, but our message is universal. We have found like-minded people who are essential to our health, and we work daily to seek gratitude and collect joy. We recommend these aspects as core elements in the journey to wellness.

At the time we were newly diagnosed, we had not met any other people in midlife with Parkinson's, especially those who were still negotiating their career or raising children. We didn't understand the importance of having supportive people around us. We were scared and unsure where to turn.

That summer, the World Parkinson Congress was held in our city, Portland Oregon. This congress is an international meeting of scientists, physicians, clinicians, caregivers, and people living with Parkinson's disease. We attended in order to better understand chronic illness and to find out what was happening to us. We wanted to hear about new therapies to treat symptoms, innovations, and most importantly, to find hope for a cure. What we sought was information, what we found was knowledge. There were nearly 5,000 people from over 23 countries attending the conference.

One hallway featured a powerful exhibit titled "This is Parkinson's" by photographer Anders Leines. The highly emotive and personal images in the exhibit showcased proud young individuals living with Parkinson's disease. Their faces reflected self-respect and humor, and we could sense that these were people who had dreams. Many were like us. Examining each of the faces in the photos brought out strong feelings of admiration and loss.

We have experienced sadness over many aspects of our illness: grief over health, grief over loss of self, grief about what we each thought aging would look like. To move on to what is, "I am a woman in midlife with Parkinson's disease," we first had to allow ourselves to grieve over how we expected our lives to be. We have found that talking with supportive friends or writing in a journal helped to guide us through the grief and ultimately to acceptance of this new life challenge. These tools, and others that we share in this book, continue to serve us well in the ongoing process of striving for wellness, and they can help you too.

REVISITING YOUR DREAMS

For much of adulthood, we are apt to put our dreams on the back burner. Productivity, independence, and achievement take center stage and are both encouraged and rewarded in our society. The focus in our lives is heavily swayed towards following the achievement path, while frivolity and daydreaming are discouraged.

The plans we had when we were young are often set aside to pursue practical routes that earn a living. However, one day we realized that this is the only life that we are given. For us, that day came with the diagnosis of Parkinson's disease. When we face a new hurdle, it is an opportunity to revisit and re-establish priorities. We are awakened to a new way of being and prompted to reevaluate our dreams.

Perhaps fairies and ballerinas are a bit far-fetched in our adult world, but we have learned to open our minds to remember our childhood dreams and find ways to incorporate them into our adult lives. We can do this in the stories we tell, the adventures we plan, and in the way, we think about ourselves. We choose to remember the magic in our childhood imaginations and the way those thoughts and dreams felt.

Now is the time to awaken those dreams and the possibilities that they offer.

At the World Parkinson Congress, we saw that opportunities still waited for us despite chronic illness. We told ourselves we would find a way in three years to attend the next one. We wanted to reconnect with this larger world and were primed for an adventure. Even the location sounded exciting: Kyoto, Japan. We had found a new dream to pursue.

Pause to reflect: *What were your dreams as a child? What did you want to be when you grew up? Are there things that you have always wanted to try or accomplish?*

Let's Do a Crazy Clap: Nancy

It is fitting that Kat and I write about our childhood dreams of fairies and ballerinas. That's the kind of kids we were, even though Kat never did see a fairy and I never got to wear a tutu. I became a lot shyer and more restrained as I got older. It was a stretch for me to become a children's librarian, but I loved being able to get down on the floor to play, imagine, and read with babies, toddlers, and three-year-olds. It was physically energetic work, and I was moving all day long, was healthy, and my body rarely felt awkward or stiff.

A highlight of being a children's librarian was working with adorably cute kids. I stamped little hands, sang nursery rhymes, waved colorful scarves, fell down, and got back up time after time to "Ring Around the Rosie." I adored being a children's librarian.

At storytime, I liked to start out with a rhyming game that began "Let's do a crazy clap." We would wave our arms high above our heads and wiggle our fingers wildly before we clapped our hands. The back of the storytime theatre had a large window, and one day I caught a glimpse of my reflection doing the crazy clap. My left arm was up high, waving, but the other arm was barely moving. Something was wrong with my right arm.

Over several weeks, I tried different stretches to unfreeze my shoulder, but the arm remained limp and slow to respond. My online searches didn't yield any results for why one arm no longer tracked the other. I was confused—and starting to worry. I felt sad at storytimes because it reminded me that something was feeling very, very wrong. I worried that I wouldn't be able to continue to do the job that I loved, and worst of all, I couldn't think of one single person in the same situation.

WHY TELLING YOUR STORY MATTERS

Stories of our childhood and thoughts about our futures and what it would be like to grow up can be a powerful guide to crafting our story as adults. People use stories to make sense of the world and to share that understanding with others. Since ancient times, spoken word and oral histories have been the way we pass down our knowledge. Our stories mark our legacy: they say we were here, we lived on this earth. Many of us can talk about a pivotal time when our lives were irrevocably changed, and we use that story to examine and illuminate the change.

The story of diagnosis often begins with how we were living a typically healthy life and then unexpectedly, we became a person living with chronic illness.

Our perception of ourselves can swiftly shift from healthy to ill, especially when confusing new things are happening in our bodies. Seeking answers to questions raised by these new things helps us make sense of and categorize our experience, and eventually contributes to treatment decisions.

Sometimes having a name to put to our symptoms can be a mental trap. We have access to abundant information, and it is easy to get lost in what could be. Having a word to describe a process, a diagnosis, can be even more detrimental to your existence if that becomes all that is defining you.

Our natural impulse to try to understand what has happened to us is powerful. We keep trying to tease out the details about how we came to be living with a brain disorder. Was it genetic? Could we have taken better care of our health? Did we deserve it somehow? We have no way of knowing why we now find ourselves in this situation.

Developing, writing, and telling our stories has helped us to accept and embrace our authentic lives, especially the difficult parts. It has helped us move from grief to compassion and to acceptance of our diagnosis. Spending reflective time thinking about what is left undone in our stories has helped inform the choices we make moving forward. Formulating the story, writing the words, and speaking the truth have all been central to accepting the reality of having a disease.

During the quarantine of 2020, we were writing our message of resilience. The tools we have learned and practiced to help us navigate our disease were the exact tools we needed to navigate the challenges of a global pandemic. Mindfulness, gratitude, and joy carried us through and became an integral part of our experience.

Stating and sharing the facts—our truths—also emboldens us to offer help to others. We hope that learning about our journey will encourage and help you to find your way. Despite a diagnosis, despite disability, despite grief and loss, despite pain, you are deserving of happiness and can train your brain to find it.

Pause to reflect: *What do you want the story of your life to be?*

Shaking and Baking: Kat

I don't remember the exact day that I was diagnosed with Parkinson's disease. I do remember the day I woke up knowing something was definitely wrong. I had been up most of the night with shaky feelings inside of my body and I realized I could not catch my breath and felt heaviness in my chest. I knew I could no longer fight off the feeling and power on through another day. Instead, I called for medical advice. I presented at urgent care where serious acute issues, like heart attack, were ruled out. I then made appointments for follow-ups with a plethora of specialists.

The reality was, I had not felt well for some time. Anxious and grieving over the death of my mother, in the midst of perimenopause, raising teenagers, working a job requiring long hours, and irregular sleep made it difficult to feel well. But the constant internal shaking feeling was a tipping point. February 4, 2015, was my last professional day—the last day of the first act of my life.

Eighteen months prior, I had accepted a promotion to director of midwifery in a large hospital-based midwifery practice. Half of my role was to lead a team of thirteen midwives in delivering care to a diverse population of women in Portland, Oregon. The other half of the role was to continue my full-scope midwifery practice. I facilitated group prenatal classes, delivered babies, saw patients in the clinic, and attended executive leadership meetings. I was invested in the practice model and in serving the women of our community.

I deeply loved my work, delivering more than 800 babies as a certified nurse midwife–nurse practitioner. I was being of service. Many of our patients had socio-cultural challenges, and I was devoted to delivering cutting-edge care. I felt at the top of my professional game even as the earliest neurologic symptoms were smoldering.

Two of our three children were grown and in college, and our youngest was soon to graduate high school. My husband was working at a stable, rewarding job. We had plans to travel to Italy to celebrate our twenty-fifth wedding anniversary. We were living our dream.

Our family had cared for my mother during her battle with cancer, losing her fight with non-Hodgkin lymphoma in the summer of 2014. Watching a person that you love suffer is gut wrenching and caring for her was physically and emotionally exhausting. I could hardly bear to watch as cancer ravaged her bones and spine, but I was a nurse practitioner and trained to take care of others, so I did.

When I was feeling off, anxious, or fatigued, I thought the grief, sleep deprivation, and perimenopausal symptoms were to blame. It would be several months before an obtuse, mat-ter-of-fact neurologist said the words "I'm fairly sure you have Parkinson's disease but come back in three months and we will confirm." All I knew was that I did not feel well, my right hand was shaking, I was suffering through hot flashes, and I felt exhausted to my absolute core.

During the time I was seeking diagnostic information, I slept up to sixteen hours a day and rarely left the house. I felt lost in a deep rabbit hole of fear, despair, and exhaustion. I felt sure that whatever it was would be short lived. I was not ready to face the possibility that I had a chronic illness.

Parkinson's was not at all on my radar, I was forty-eight years old, far too young, or so I thought. My father and two uncles had Parkinson's disease, but neither were diagnosed before the age of sixty. As a clinician, I had studied the neurologic system and was intimately familiar with symptoms, but not for a middle-aged woman, not for me.

Once confirmed months later, the diagnosis did not come as a surprise. My husband and I went to my follow-up appointment more equipped with questions and information. The words were then spoken: "You have young-onset Parkinson's disease." The neurologist's advice was to go on and live your life. Great advice, but how do I do that?

Maybe humor was a good start, so I decided I would share with friends and family that I was shaking and baking my way through mid-life.

Meet Our Friend: Michelle

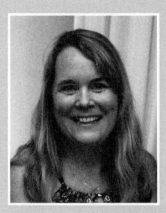

Ever wonder where that sultry jazz singer with the honey rich sound is today? We know! We met her when she first came to our boxing class. Michelle was a jazz singer in the hip Southern California beach clubs in the eighties and later went on to raise a family and teach preschool. She was diagnosed with Parkinson's at the age of forty-nine, after being misdiagnosed twice. Her father also lives with Parkinson's disease after being diagnosed in his seventies.

Michelle stopped working in her beloved preschool classroom when she became worried that her balance might cause her to injure a child should she trip. Stiffness in her hands was making it hard to help the children do art and coordination difficulties complicated her effort to keep rhythm to the beat of her music lessons.

When she could no longer work, Michelle decided to return to singing, her first love. She learned about the voice challenges faced by people with Parkinson's disease and offers classes with our local nonprofit groups serving people with the disease. Best of all, she still has that honey rich sound. ❋

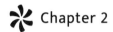 Chapter 2

THE WELLNESS SPIRAL

"We are not going in circles, we are going upwards. The path
is a spiral; we have already climbed many steps."

—HERMANN HESSE

WE HAVE LEARNED A lot since the first days of our diagnoses and have come to see the journey to wellness as an upward spiral. Our wellness spiral is a useful model for visualizing the path ahead whenever you face a life event or pivotal time, such as a diagnosis of chronic illness or find yourself feeling emotions such as anxiety or despair.

The wellness spiral provides a framework for movement. You can navigate along the spiral, sometimes moving up and sometimes down, and you can linger where you need to. In this chapter and in further reading throughout the rest of this book, we will provide more information about the spiral, and how to use it. Moving along the spiral takes the ability to change and adapt, and the capacity to recover from difficulties. Elasticity gives you the ability to spring back and is determined by how resilient you are.

A key component to wellness is being able to move forward even when presented with challenges or obstacles. All of our lives are a compilation of experiences. We are all resilient and hold the ability to be well. Resilience, the ability to thrive despite adversity, helps us to navigate our lives and allows for growth and expansive opportunity. With intention, it will also keep us from identifying solely as ill, sick, or disabled.

Historically, a spiral has signified movement, growth, opportunity, and sometimes the sacred. It is a common petroglyphic symbol found carved onto ancient stones. Our spiral starts out small and winding and then moves up and outward to an expanse of wide-open possibility. The spiral leads upward to intentional wellness, which encompasses overall health and well-being. It incorporates the steps along the spiral: treating yourself and others with compassion, building community, and developing a practice of gratitude. Movement along the spiral is not sequential or fixed, but rather a fluid process.

We created the wellness spiral after being introduced to an advocacy pyramid as envisioned by the late Parkinson's advocate Tom Isaacs, and the researcher Dr. Sonia Mather. Their advocacy pyramid starts with a diagnosis and ends with a cure (Isaacs, 2015). Although our models are very different, the spiral explores a similar pathway, in our case, to find wellness after the disruption of a major life event.

One of our favorite steps along the spiral is joy and contentment. You may notice that we use the word joy often. We feel strongly about seeking it in our own lives and hope to guide you to cultivate more in your own. We value joy so much we included the following definition. Delight, gaiety, bliss…what's not to like?

joy **noun**

\ ˈjȯi \

Definition of *joy*

1 a : emotion evoked by well-being, success, or good fortune or by the prospect of possessing what one desires: DELIGHT

  b : the expression or exhibition of such emotion: GAIETY

2 : a state of happiness or felicity: BLISS

3 : a source or cause of delight

THE SPIRAL

Even when living with challenges, one can be well. We do not mean to say that we never feel down or worried. Negative thoughts can sneak in, and grief is an important and necessary step in accepting a diagnosis. However, by practicing the methods we describe here, we are building the pathways in our brains that can lead us out of despair.

Despite our diagnoses, a goal of wellness guides the way we live, think, and see our futures. We created the illustration of the wellness spiral to serve as a visual reminder of how you can take active steps in training your brain to find gratitude for all that you have. The spiral represents the expanse of possibility. It is adaptable and allows movement into and out of the various stages as one works from diagnosis and grief toward healing. We do not graduate from one stage, never to return. We constantly keep moving along our journey to find resilience and joy, no matter the challenge.

Many types of wellness exist including physical, mental, spiritual, intellectual, and metaphysical. In our model, we focus on intentionally choosing to be well and on defining ourselves as well. Each part of the spiral you travel contains unique aspects relevant to your circumstances.

Along the spiral are a number of steps on which you can land. Each step is a particular manifestation of the current state of wellness that you are experiencing. The steps don't just happen on their own; rather, it takes action and thought to arrive at a new step. Flowing from the bottom to the top, the spiral has the following steps:

THE WELLNESS SPIRAL

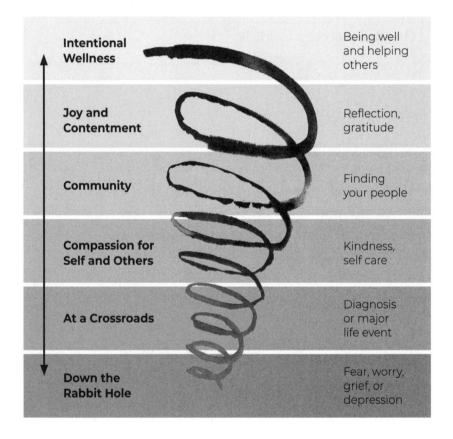

Intentional Wellness	Being well and helping others
Joy and Contentment	Reflection, gratitude
Community	Finding your people
Compassion for Self and Others	Kindness, self care
At a Crossroads	Diagnosis or major life event
Down the Rabbit Hole	Fear, worry, grief, or depression

Rabbit hole. A spiral flows both up and down. The tight, small end of our spiral represents burrowing into a hole. We use the term rabbit hole to represent a place with negative thoughts under the surface that are hard to escape. Rabbit holes disrupt the wellness process. Without respite, rabbit hole thinking can lead to catastrophizing, depression, and more.

When you have a chronic, incurable disease, it is easy to get lost in thoughts of its progression and the "what ifs." The internet is plagued with examples of disabling symptoms, and this kind of thinking centers around disability, disease, and disaster, and can cause despair. Other examples of rabbit hole thinking are circular thinking, perseverating, worry, anxiety, and grief.

If our only thoughts are of despair, those are the primary reactions our brain allows. Teaching ourselves to stay out of the rabbit hole allows us to find the expanse of intentional wellness. The more we think about compassion, joy, and gratitude, the less room there is for the paths of thought that loop into the rabbit hole. The pathways take up space that may have been occupied by rabbit-hole thinking.

Each time you successfully find your way out of a rabbit hole pattern, a path is created to follow more easily the next time.

Diagnosis or major life event / At a crossroads. This is a decision point. Some examples of crossroad events are death, marriage, divorce, illness, retirement, a new job, a layoff at work, or a move. The crossroads stage can be a time of great uncertainty.

Major life events can be extremely complicated, and you may want to break them down into smaller categories or decision points to help you better understand how you want to move forward.

Compassion. A strong feeling of caring, particularly for yourself and your own well-being, can be a positive first step of movement up the spiral after a life event occurs. This compassion step is the time and place for practicing kind self-talk, particularly about life acceptance (both the good and bad). Other ways to express compassion are loving yourself, forgiving transgressions, forgiving others, integrating all parts of self, seeing potential in yourself and others, and focusing on abilities.

Community. The people in your life form your community, and they often come from your neighborhood, family, family of choice, church, exercise class and similar activities, and other like-minded folks. Research shows us the importance of intentionally building a sense of community and finding who makes you feel good.

Joy and contentment. Actively seeking happiness, fulfillment, and contentmentis a key component in achieving wellness. Writing the moments down, taking photos, sketching, producing art and music can all help to capture and document the joyful moments. This step includes recognizing joy, looking for it, planning for it, respecting it, and intentionally finding time to spend with others who seek joy.

Intentional wellness. Finding the right balance for you of all the wellness components. Some examples are telling your story, allowing space to be seen and heard by others, and taking comfort in self. Little time is spent in rabbit-hole thinking and more time is spent building community, writing, speaking, and helping others to share their stories. When moments of despair creep in, it is easy to refocus and return to positive thinking. At this step, you are maximizing the time spent feeling well and joyful.

Pause to reflect: *How does the spiral resonate with you? Which aspects call to you to work on? Consider jotting down a few thoughts about where you will start.*

GRIEF

Even though it is not officially part of the wellness spiral, we want to acknowledge how important grieving is to achieving wellness. Once you are able to grieve, you can begin to start understanding your diagnosis. Be kind to yourself and take your time. A diagnosis—like any major life event—brings us to a crossroads. With upheaval and grief, there can be a great opportunity for creation and a fresh start.

Tuning into your body is a way to start practicing reflection. In our fast-paced society, we are just learning the importance of slowing down. Sometimes with a diagnosis, we get a nudge to put the brakes on. There are times we must be quiet in the barrage of chaos around us to take a moment to look within to hear ourselves.

Now is the time for being. It may be the beginning of an era of less doing. Make "to be" lists instead of "to do" lists. Slowing down from a hectic pace of life can be healing. The world experienced an unprecedented change of pace during the quarantine in 2020, much like how Parkinson's slows us down. It makes sure our body lets us know if we are doing too much of some things and not enough of others.

The Kubler-Ross studies pose a model for understanding grief. These studies were conducted with terminally ill people or those who had recently lost a loved one and described the process of grief. Their work has been widely accepted as a model for grieving in general. They define specific steps that we move through as we grieve loss. You likely have heard of these: denial, anger, bargaining, depression, and acceptance. These are not linear steps; you don't finish one then move onto the next never to return. They are processes that one will move in and out of as they go through the grieving process.

Like the Kubler-Ross model of grief, we believe that you can follow a similar path to wellness. After receiving news of a diagnosis and grieving, you can achieve a state of chronic wellness. It is a different way to view wellness and illness and allows for both. Our spiral accepts diagnosis and grieving as part of a process that ultimately builds to joy and contentment and like the Kubler-Ross model you may move in and out of aspects of the spiral over time.

Dr. Cecilia Chan and her colleagues studied how spiritual practice may impact coping after experiencing a major life event. They studied how people who practice Eastern religions cope with grief versus those that did not identify a spiritual practice. A key aspect in those that showed more resilience was the ability to distinguish the difference between having control over life choices in response to the life event versus perceived control over the actual event. Those who practiced eastern religion accepted more readily that they did not have control over these events and in general, coped better.

Pause to reflect: *How will you incorporate all that came before your diagnosis but is now different? Start to pay attention to the things that make you sad and also the things that make you feel good (the things that make you smile and bring a sense of wonder, curiosity, or contentment).*

THE ROLE OF RESILIENCE

We all come into this day with a brain full of tools that help us to get through our lives. We have inherent knowledge, strength, and resilience or we would not have made it this far. Resilience helps us to navigate our journey along the wellness spiral and keeps us from getting lost in rabbit-hole thinking. Some of us have more life experiences that help lay the foundation for integrating a new challenge. For others, it is all new. Our stories, our experiences of resilience, and the words we tell ourselves and others will inform how we navigate a new challenge.

Flowers and Daisies: Kat

Much of what I know of resilience, I learned from our family, and it served me well as I grappled with my diagnosis. Sawyer, the youngest of our three children, had just turned eight when he was diagnosed with type 1 diabetes, and life as we knew it was forever changed.

Because his pancreas fails to make the insulin he needs to live, our family learned how to give him insulin. We learned to count every carbohydrate, calculate carb-to-insulin ratios, and how to stick a finger to test his blood. The days blurred with a series of tests followed by injections. His fingers became calloused, his body bruised by injections. As his mother, I begged the universe to let us trade places. He deserved a healthy, carefree childhood. It might have been easy to fall into the rabbit hole and stay in fear and worry, and hyper focusing on his illness.

We chose to accept the challenges of managing his disease while working and encouraging our children to live active and engaged lives. My husband, our three children, and I, juggled blood-sugar testing, insulin dosing, swim meets, scout meetings, soccer games, running a small business, and keeping a private midwifery practice thriving. We met other diabetic families through a summer camp program and found joy in family dinners, camping trips, and holiday celebrations.

I told myself, "At least I am a health care professional and know about the disease," and "I was trained for this." No one can ever train you to watch your child endure the management of a lifelong chronic disease. I felt the drain of feeling responsible for Sawyer's disease management and his response to his "new normal" life. I carried a pager for my work and for Sawyer.

Our family was learning about resilience while Sawyer learned how to coexist with a chronic disease. He could choose to be known by and defined by his disease or focus on all of his other wonderful qualities. I am grateful he chose the latter.

Several months into the diagnosis Sawyer stated matter-of-factly, "Mom, you give horrible injections!"

"What? I am a trained professional!" I replied.

"I want to give my own shots," he asserted.

Was it all right to let an eight-year-old do this? After a discussion, he learned how to give himself shots. From that day forward, we only gave injections in the middle of the night.

One day I noticed him mumbling to himself before injecting his insulin. It looked like he was coaching himself. With tears in my eyes, I asked if he was scared about it hurting. After finishing his injection, he turned to me and held my hands.

He looked sympathetically into my teary eyes and said, "Don't worry Mama, all I have to do is think about flowers and daisies and it is all ok." His strategy immediately allayed my worries and was a powerful testament to his strength and resilience.

It has been nearly two decades since Sawyer's diagnosis. We have learned a great deal about resilience as a family. Ken and I have worked to keep our lines of communication open and honest about pressures, joys, limits, and personal desires. We have been held up in times of crisis by our community and our family has learned to accept illness as a part of life while not being defined by it.

We cherish our marriage and feel that we are stronger for all we have navigated together. Communication and slow dancing in our kitchen whenever the mood strikes are our secrets to making it work. Whether dealing with diabetes, Parkinson's disease, cancer, crooked teeth, or a bad hair day, we have a choice about our attitude. Challenges can define us, or we can think of flowers and daisies and put one foot in front of the other.

When I was diagnosed with Parkinson's disease, I felt like I had a familiar framework for organizing my thoughts and reactions. I knew from the beginning that I would not choose to be defined by my diagnosis, but I did need to learn a new way to be me with Parkinson's disease.

Being resilient doesn't mean that you never experience difficulty or distress. It is the ability to adapt in the face of adversity. Resilience helps you recover and trains your brain to do it again when needed.

On a Mountain High: Nancy

My route to becoming resilient was never straightforward. For many years, I wandered in circles and often lost my way. I didn't always plan to be a librarian, and I worked instead as a technical writer. By the time I was in my late thirties, I was single, restless, and knew that I didn't want to be an employee of a stuffy corporation. Everything about my life felt stressful, particularly the work pressure.

Recent research shows Parkinson's disease starts many years before the onset of motor symptoms and may even occur before birth. If this is true, I was already starting to experience cell loss in the brain related to Parkinson's disease. I was aware of none of this. I just had a strong urge to change my life.

I changed it in the best way I could. I had read about a small organization doing hawk migration research, and I set off with a tent and sleeping bag to join them. We made our base camp high in the Manzano Mountains outside of Albuquerque. There was no electricity or running water. At night the stars were brilliant, and I fell asleep to owls calling. I slept easily with no signs of the Parkinson's symptoms that would come much later in my life. Every morning I hiked two to three miles in rugged terrain to get to my research station. My legs and body became stronger. I was fifteen years older than most of my camp mates, and some days I struggled with being slower and weaker than the young men and women in their twenties.

Still, the Manzanos were spectacular. I worked hard and fell into the habit of ending my day sitting on a rock outcrop, feeling inspired by the wilderness and so very lucky to be there. This is where I first practiced mindfulness. I learned to be still, and it was then that I knew that I could handle whatever came my way. This knowledge has stayed with me over the years and is invaluable when I am struggling.

In the mountains, I felt alive in my body and my mind was sharp, but I know now that the seeds of Parkinson's were likely already germinating.

The weather turned colder. The work became harder. Then an interesting thing happened. One by one, my younger camp mates started to leave. Our numbers dwindled. And still, there I was, a tortoise in the race, an elder, one still standing. I withstood the storm and, in the process, learned to be steady and calm and strong.

Never again would I need proof of what I could accomplish. I learned everything I needed to know about resilience on a mountain high in the Manzanos.

GETTING STARTED

Learning to live with a chronic illness can awaken your inner strength, and prompt you to dig deep and learn about yourself in new ways. Soon you will share your own story of resilience.

Most of us have had challenging experiences and have learned from them. No one that we have met has gotten far in life without encountering unexpected difficulties or suffering. Paying attention and being present in the world can help you to build resilience and learn from your experiences.

Look at the wellness spiral earlier in this chapter and think about a challenging time in your life. Reflect on how you managed it.

If your pace today is so hectic that you cannot pause, reflect, and integrate experiences as they happen, it may be wise to re-evaluate your pace. Can you add regular time for quiet reflection? Being present and in the moment carries opportunities to find joy and wellness as you travel your path.

Your answers can help to guide you through challenges. Do not be afraid of reflecting back and recognizing what you have learned. We suspect you will find many examples of your strength and resilience on the path to intentional wellness.

Meet Our Friend: Jane

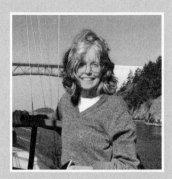

She is stunning on the ballroom dance floor. As you watch Jane's elegant twirls you would never guess the obstacles she has overcome. Diagnosed with Parkinson's at age fifty-two, Jane felt the stressors of her MBA work and full-time job at a large publishing house exacerbate her symptoms.

In a defining life moment, Jane made a dramatic decision to follow her dreams. She and her boyfriend sailed the Pacific north to Alaska and back, then began to plot a course around the world.

Her dream was cut short when she fell on the sailboat, suffering major facial and head trauma. She lost her right eye. Seven months later she developed a rare autoimmune condition that attacked her left eye, threatening to leave her blind. Around this time, her boyfriend broke off their relationship.

Through it all—Parkinson's, the fall, threat of blindness, becoming unexpectedly single, Jane found remarkable resilience. She began learning ballroom dance and participated in competitions across the country. She inspires us with her grace and ready smile. And whenever the music begins, Jane leads us out on the floor to dance. ✳

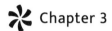 Chapter 3

THE RABBIT HOLE

"Lean forward into your life: Begin each day as if it were on purpose."

—MARY ANNE RADMACHER

IN LEWIS CARROLL'S BOOK *Alice's Adventures in Wonderland*, Alice falls down a rabbit hole and enters a strange and unsettling place. Similarly, the rabbit hole of chronic illness is a state of mind into which any of us can tumble. We fall into despair or depression, or we start feeling anxious or numb. Once we are in a rabbit hole, we often neglect our health and our friends, and like Alice, we cannot easily find a way back out.

The rabbit hole lies at the bottom of the spiral. You can find yourself in a deep emotional hole seemingly without warning. When you are in that rabbit hole, it feels like it takes more effort to climb out than you can manage. Getting out of a rabbit hole requires work and making a commitment to balancing different aspects of good health.

Not everyone experiences the rabbit hole in the same way, but few in life get by without encountering some difficulties. No matter how prepared you are, it is nothing short of life-changing to hear you have a progressive, incurable illness. Each of us reacts in our own way, and most of us need time and support to sort it out. We have shared a lot of tears with newly diagnosed people over fears about what the future might hold. With a little time, the diagnosis becomes a lot less scary for most people.

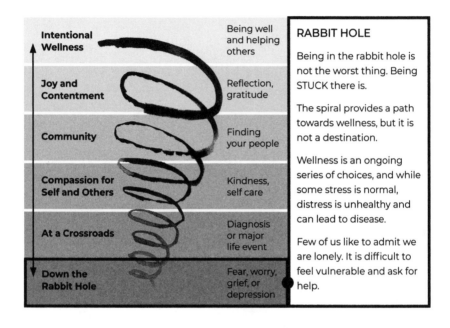

		RABBIT HOLE
Intentional Wellness	Being well and helping others	Being in the rabbit hole is not the worst thing. Being STUCK there is.
Joy and Contentment	Reflection, gratitude	The spiral provides a path towards wellness, but it is not a destination.
Community	Finding your people	
Compassion for Self and Others	Kindness, self care	Wellness is an ongoing series of choices, and while some stress is normal, distress is unhealthy and can lead to disease.
At a Crossroads	Diagnosis or major life event	
Down the Rabbit Hole	Fear, worry, grief, or depression	Few of us like to admit we are lonely. It is difficult to feel vulnerable and ask for help.

We found it hopeful to learn that although Parkinson's moves at different paces for different people, changes tend to come on slowly. It is impossible to know which symptoms you may develop, you can't predict how they will impact your life, and you can't know how quickly they will progress. Each of us has a unique journey with many paths to choose along the way.

When you feel stuck in a difficult place, it is often hard to find a way forward. We all wish it were as easy as finding a hidden door or a magical potion. Just like Alice learned in her Wonderland, the path ahead is not always simple to follow. We believe, and the research supports, that with practice and intention you can train yourself to avoid the deepest rabbit holes more quickly and easily. We also believe there is something to be learned from being stuck. If we never experience hardship or sadness, we also miss out on joy.

MENTAL HEALTH

According to the National Institute of Health, one of five adults in the United States live with a mental illness and it is estimated that only half receive treatment for it. During the pandemic, these rates were even higher. Many who have Parkinson's disease struggle with depression and anxiety. In fact, people with Parkinson's are more likely to develop these mental health conditions than the rest of the population. For some, mental health problems precede their Parkinson's diagnosis by many years (Giroux and Farris, 2019).

In order to find wellness, it is crucial that we take care of our whole selves, including our mental health. That means paying attention to our mental state, recognizing if and when we need help, and following the advice of a doctor or other medical professional. Common treatments for mild to moderate depression and anxiety include exercise, counseling, and medication.

Choosing to face depression and anxiety and finding ways to manage the symptoms can be the difference between simply settling for getting by, versus finding meaning and enjoyment in your life. Many can and do survive lifetimes with anxiety and depression, but wouldn't it be nice to thrive, not just merely get by? It is yet another choice in how we manage our lives and choose our paths.

The Neurotransmitter Dance

It is useful to know a little bit about what is going awry in your body when you have a chronic illness in order to understand how you might best cope with the changes. Our bodies are complex systems that rely on a balance of many elements, including neurotransmitters which act as the body's chemical messengers. They are the molecules used by the nervous system to transmit messages between neurons, or from neurons to muscles.

Neurotransmitters are part of what enables our nervous system to function properly. An imbalance or lack of production can impact many body functions. Though not completely understood, it is suspected that these imbalances can cause disease. The goal with treatment is to encourage activities that will enhance production or usage of the existing amounts that the body produced or to supplement a deficiency. (Johns Hopkins Medicine, 2021)

Dopamine is a neurotransmitter that helps muscles move. People with Parkinson's disease do not make enough dopamine due to damage to the cells that make dopamine. Tremors, bradykinesia (slow movement), muscle weakness, and cramping can all be related to lack of dopamine. For each person with Parkinson's, symptoms will manifest differently. Parkinson's is a fascinating disease (although a little less fascinating when you are experiencing it yourself). Not knowing what symptoms you may face and how to predict a solution can be frustrating for the person with Parkinson's, their care partners, and health care providers.

Some neurotransmitters help us to feel good and experience happiness. Dopamine is one of these. We also produce serotonin when we feel love and joy. For people struggling with depression, accessing the body's serotonin levels may be more difficult. Therefore, activities to enhance serotonin levels such as exercise and medications often help enhance and stabilize these levels. Medications can also help the nervous system be more efficient at using the serotonin that is produced.

It makes sense that science finds that people diagnosed with Parkinson's disease have neurotransmitters that are out of balance. This can explain many symptoms, muscle impairments, and mental health. The same is speculated about the imbalance of serotonin in those with depression.

STRESS

It can be difficult to manage the many demands of daily life, family, and self-care in the smoothest of times, but success in these areas can make a significant difference to your health and well-being. Achieving some control over stress is essential. Otherwise, the pull itself becomes a source of ongoing stress.

We know that life will not exist without stress. Some is necessary, but too much stress, or distress, is detrimental. Distress can show up as shortness of breath, muscle tension, neck and back pain, trouble sleeping, change in appetite, or loss of interest in our usual pleasures, to name just a few possibilities. When we experience these symptoms, our body is signaling to us that we have exceeded its tolerance for how we are functioning or trying to function.

In a stress response, we produce cortisol, and our sympathetic nervous system's fight or flight response is activated. Historically, this state allowed for us to focus our energy on the central parts of our bodies, diverting blood from non-vital functions such as digestion to aid our large muscles that may need to help us run. Our pupils dilate and allow our focus to be sharp. If a predator was after us, we could run and escape, using the muscles needed to get away.

This adaptation served us well when we might have been preyed upon. However, in our modern world, this response tends to be overactivated and we stay hyper-alert too much of the time. Learning to move out of a stress response and to temper cortisol production can move us towards a state of well-being—or balance—and out of distress. This, of course, is easier said than done, and finding balance can be as elusive as it is imperative.

Here are some ways to reduce stress:

- Relax using yoga or meditation, maybe try a new app

- Take a low intensity walk, a stroll. Stop and admire the view

- Get a hug from a good friend

- Reassess your to-do list and cross a few things off

- Listen to or play low-stress music

Many factors can predict how we deal with stress. Our personality, our resources, our histories, and our health all contribute to stress management. In fact, evidence suggests that our belief in our own abilities affects our coping skills. The Social Readjustment Rating Scale (SRRS) developed in the late 1960s by two psychiatrists is one way to describe how self-confidence can impact wellness. Researchers studied two groups of people: one group reported that they got ill after experiencing a high stress event while the other reported remaining healthy after such an event. Those who remained healthy during high stress times scored higher self-esteem than the other group did. (Holmes & Rahe, 1967)

Self-esteem is important to our mental health. Though researchers debate whether low self-esteem contributes to depression or if depression erodes self-esteem, they agree that the two are strongly related (Sowislo & Orth, 2013). Activities that enhance our sense of worth and well-being are critically linked to our mental health.

When there is a new physiological challenge like Parkinson's disease, it is a time to evaluate how to maximize healthy options and self-confidence and minimize those things in our lives that may contribute to or hasten our disease. Health care experts encourage us to reduce stress, which takes self-awareness and practice to achieve. Reducing stress may be the single most important way to contribute to our well-being.

The Fixers

A unique type of stress comes from people who appear to have good intentions. They want to tell us all the details of another new cure for Parkinson's disease that they read about online or in a magazine. It's not a medical cure and it's not backed by any doctors or medical journals. Suddenly our calm demeanor flies out the window, and the skies turn stormy. Our reduced-stress day is waylaid.

We call these people "the fixers." We try to steer a clear path away from them, or at least their fixes. They'll ask, "Have you tried this special diet supplement?" and we work to not interpret the question as intrusive or a form of judgment. If you want to get better, we imagine they are thinking, why aren't you doing this, or trying that? As our friend Kerry Rae likes to say, "I'd love to hear from you, but please don't give me advice."

We are doing everything we know how to do. We have probably already read the research about the special diet supplement, or we talked to our doctor and got a thumbs down. We are open to new ideas, but we try to make up our minds based on current credible research. When it comes to disease, we all wish we could fix what cannot be fixed.

The fixers are drawn to social media like moths. If you post an update on your health, you are likely to get a fixer comment. "Have you tried eating [something like organic alfalfa]?" they'll ask innocently. "My uncle eats [organic alfalfa] and now he's almost completely cured." You might also encounter a do-gooder that will lead into their advice with "my uncle's cousin's best friend's niece is a doctor, and she recommends..." You get the picture. Unsolicited advice from essentially unknown sources is most often not worth considering.

We would like to mention those that claim to have cured their incurable disease. There can be those that have built their entire life around minimizing symptoms that they wish to "sell" to you as a cure. We have yet to find any cure, free, prescribed, or written about. We advise you to act on advice from your team before buying into any expensive program or a new treatment claiming to fix all.

Parkinson's disease presents and develops very differently for different people. Progression is unique for everyone, as is life. Sometimes we want so badly to explain what is happening to our bodies and the progression of symptoms that we blame ourselves or our loved ones or care partners when we notice something new. We may be tempted to blame ourselves. Don't. No one needs to feel judged for a process that largely cannot be controlled.

If a cure is found, we think the medical community will be very interested in hearing about it. It won't just be advertised on social media. There will be large-scale verification trials set up. Neurologists will tell us about it. We aren't worried about missing the news because it will be everywhere.

ISOLATION AND LONELINESS

Many of us have known the pain of feeling lonely. Researchers have now shown that being isolated from others can have very real consequences. When we lack social connections, it significantly increases our risk of having health problems, even more than commonly recognized hazards such as obesity, physical inactivity, air pollution, or smoking cigarettes (Holt-Lunstad, 2017).

Sometimes, in the depths of pain and sadness, it takes all of one's energy to connect. Planning to meet others and honoring commitments keeps us going. Many people are more reliable if they make a commitment to another person to attend a class or meet up.

Seeking out a professional counselor can relieve the feeling that we are burdening our loved ones with our discussions about our process. For some care partners, it can be stressful to be the only confidants to loved ones living with a chronic illness. Trained therapists are alert to the signs and symptoms of depression and anxiety and can help with tools to treat and maximize mental health. They typically are not licensed to manage prescription medications but can help to decide when it may be time to consider medication or a change in prescription.

Sometimes it is helpful to have a safe place to process our fears that we may not want to share with anyone else in our family. Having a prescribed time, place, and person whose only role is to listen and guide is a comforting complement to our team of providers.

Chronic illness can provide a renewed opportunity to connect to people in our lives and make choices about how we wish to live. Priorities start to become clear by the actions we take, and how we spend our time and energy with people in our life. We explore more about the importance of building a supportive group of friends in the pages ahead.

Pause to reflect: *Consider writing about three things that make you feel stressed or lonely. Then follow with three things that you like about yourself, such as your energy, compassion, or kindness. Were you able to shift your focus?*

MINDFULNESS

Developing a mindfulness practice can be a path out of the rabbit hole. Mindfulness is defined as being fully present in the moment, thinking only of the now, not the past or the future. Many people practice mindfulness using meditation, yoga, or deep breathing. We have learned to practice mindfulness through some of these methods. As our bodies have changed, we have learned to slow our minds down and enjoy our moments.

The health benefits of meditation and yoga are well-documented. A regular meditation practice can lower blood pressure and calm the sympathetic nervous system (our fight or flight response). Taking deep, slow breaths can have similar calming effects. Yoga combines meditative breathing with the added benefits of strengthening muscles and aiding balance. These are not new discoveries; they have been around and practiced by many cultures for centuries.

For those of us with a neurologic disease, it is important to find ways to better understand how our own system works. We need to figure out how to give ourselves more conscious attention to foster well-being.

It's easy to disconnect our thoughts from the way that we are feeling in our bodies and emotions. However, disengaging isn't a healthy way to live. It means that we are ignoring the signals that our bodies are sending to get our attention. We might be denying that our stomach is too full or that it is complaining about a rich diet. We can ignore the signs that we are not getting enough sleep or exercise, that our necks hurt because we are tense and using poor posture, or that we are stuffing our feelings down so that we do not act sad or angry, or jealous. It is often valued in our fast-paced world to "buck up" or "power through" even when feeling poorly.

If that sounds familiar to you, then mindfulness practice can help you become more in touch with your body and better able to cope with the stress of a chronic disease. Mindfulness can be practiced either inside or outside of meditation and is often centered on the breath. You can try it out by taking three or four breaths and paying attention to how the breath feels to you as it comes in and out of your body. That action is mindfulness in one of its simplest forms.

You can practice mindfulness just about anywhere. Whenever you are breathing, you can do it with mindfulness. The key is to be present and in the moment. It may take a little time to get accustomed to focusing on your breath, but it will come a little more naturally to you soon enough.

Some people practice by taking themselves to a special place in their mind. This might be a sunny beach, a mountain retreat, or a favorite chair. Wherever that relaxing, comforting, calming space is for you, use it as a leaping off place. Perhaps the place is tied to a favorite memory, a time of serenity and contentment.

What other memories evoke joy, or a deep sense of well-being? A family vacation? A trip to a favorite family member? A hike or camp out? Make this a place that you can visit anytime you wish, in your mind. An easy way to get started is to close your eyes and picture what you see in a place that you would love to be. Can you feel the sun on your face? What sounds do you hear? Remember all the sensations you can. Know that at any time you can return to this place and this sense of peace and calm.

A practice of any sort must be repeated. Habits develop with consistency. If you can repeat a practice for several weeks, it becomes a habit. It may help to integrate your mindfulness practice into your existing schedule by pairing it with another task or as part of your routine.

I Am One Human Being Doing the Best That I Can: Kat

It was a particularly busy time in my life with three children at home, working as a midwife in a busy private practice, and being on call. This meant seeing patients in the office and managing patients in the hospital fifty percent of all hours. Babies come when they are ready. As a midwife, under low-risk circumstances, I was trained to trust the physiological process of labor and the wisdom and strength that women possess, while keeping a watchful eye out for complications. For a midwife, this means spending a great deal of time awake all hours of the day and night watchfully supporting and allowing the process of birth to unfold.

It was during this time that I learned to meditate. I felt stuck in an unrelenting place of anxiety, a rabbit hole. I needed relief and thought I might try meditation. To be entirely honest, I never thought myself capable of clearing my mind. Truth be told, I have never succeeded at it completely, but what I tried did help.

I started my practice slowly in the shower. It was a private place that was comforting and soothing. It was quiet and I could be alone and focus. I would sit in the bathtub and allow the shower to rain down. I would close my eyes and breathe deeply (just like I would coach my patients to do). On the "in" breath I would focus on the word peace (peace for myself, peace for my family, for my friends, for my patients, for the world). With each deep inhalation, I would send my small message of peace to others. When I exhaled, I would do the same with the message of love. At the start, I did this for about five minutes.

At the end of each "session" or shower, I would focus on the sentence, "I am one human being doing the best that I can." Not a profound statement or a worldly tribute to a time-honored deity, rather a self-compassionate statement that worked for me. I felt calm and more equipped to face the demands of the day ahead. I became better at quieting my mind and slowly worked up to doing about fifteen minutes during my morning routine. Maybe you can find a simple way to start a practice that helps you. Try adding deep breaths to your shower routine and see how it makes you feel. You might add a phrase that reinforces all that you are in the world.

Even on a Crowded Bus: Nancy

Each day, we see reasons to feel depressed or anxious, and this leads to the kind of thinking that puts us in a rabbit hole. I learned to combat those feelings by practicing mindfulness on my daily bus commute. It might sound impossible to do with other people around, but it is not at all. I know several people who regularly listen to recorded guided mindfulness exercises on their commute, or they meditate while they sit quietly in a back hall or empty office.

I start by taking a few deep breaths. I check my posture. Are my shoulders down and back? Am I holding my core muscles so that they support me? Is my head up? I close my eyes, take a few more calming breaths, and return my thoughts gently, over, and over, to the present moment. I sit quietly, ever mindful of my place in the big world.

Sometimes I hear nearby conversations, or an announcement, "Next stop, Morrison Bridge," and sometimes I just hear the hum of the bus in motion. I let the sounds wash through me without lingering, and I arrive feeling focused and present.

REFRAMING

In an already tough time, we start the spinning downward spiral of catastrophizing our lives. We all have been here at one time or another. It is a spin that, if left unattended, can result in unrelenting dread and fear. Here we describe a specific way that you might get yourself out of the rabbit hole way of thinking by rephrasing.

For those of us with Parkinson's disease, a rabbit hole spiral might sound something like this. "I feel too tired to go exercise today." "I am so much more tired with Parkinson's." "Nothing seems to help this." "It is only going to get worse." "It's incurable." "I'm just not going to put out the effort to go exercise anymore." "What's the point?"

Our minds will take us down, but they can also be trained to steer us out of the spiral. "I feel too tired to exercise today." "I am so much more tired with Parkinson's." These are cues that the brain needs redirection. "Exercise is my medicine to slow down my disease." "I often feel more energy after I exercise." "I am going to work out and rest afterward if I am still tired."

WAITING FOR A CURE

Part of having an incurable illness is the obvious interest in a cure. We would all welcome a world with less disease and suffering. However, becoming overly invested in looking for a cure can be disappointing and difficult. Many people that we have met with a chronic illness talk of what they will do when a cure is found. There are hundreds of studies and promising research at every turn for so many diseases. However, we have a choice regarding where we put our time and energy, what we read, what we search for online, and what we subscribe to. To invest hope in every promising study means time spent not investing in the present. Do not put off finding your joy. Focusing on what might happen can be a rabbit hole, of sorts, that puts off focusing on the current day or being mindful.

So far, all of the promising studies have not found the answer and the reality is that many more studies are likely to fail before we have a cure for Parkinson's. We are in no way discouraging you from participating in research. We must help to move science forward. A healthy balance is the key to contributing to research while maintaining overall health.

Sawyer Waits: Kat

After Sawyer's diagnosis, we followed research about diabetes. His physician shared that she thought a cure was close and would be found in his lifetime and we clung to that. Sawyer would get excited to hear about results that seemed promising, and we would discuss them feeling hopeful. Then as studies progressed and were found to be inconclusive or unhelpful, he would get sad and discouraged. It became a rollercoaster ride for us, so we decided to change our approach.

We didn't stop wishing for a cure; rather, we decided to focus on the things we could control. We discontinued notifications of new studies and limited how often we followed research progress, checking quarterly before Sawyer's endocrinology visits. We stopped looking to the future to find happiness and became more present in the now once we let go of the constant search for the cure.

Meet Our Friend: **Karen**

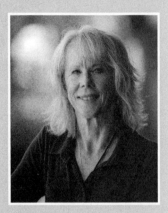

We noticed a beautiful lavender tattoo on Karen's ankle at our early morning boxing bootcamp. The tattoo commemorates her only child, Sadie, who Karen and her husband lost to depression and suicide when Sadie was 18.

Karen was diagnosed with Parkinson's disease in her early sixties. She is also a cancer survivor. Despite these challenges, hers is a story of hope. Karen is resilient and continues to search for positive ways to work through her loss and grief. She is the author of a beautiful book about Sadie's life, *Searching for Normal: The Story of a Girl Gone Too Soon*, which includes excerpts from Sadie's poetry and other writings.

Karen is a warm and quiet woman made of steel. She is an avid traveler, cyclist, and pickleball player. In Sadie's absence, Karen provides guidance and resources to families and is an advocate for struggling youth who need community, awareness, and most of all, hope. ✳

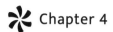 Chapter 4

CROSSROADS

"Let yourself be silently drawn by the strange pull of what you really love. It will not lead you astray."

—RUMI

THE LIFE CHANGING DIAGNOSIS of a chronic illness can bring up unexpected emotions. You may feel overwhelmed, or numb, or even as if you have taken a physical blow to your body. The force of the diagnosis can feel so strong that you wonder how you will be able to keep going forward. You may experience the same feelings when you go through other life experiences. We identify these life events as *crossroads*. When at a crossroads, if we have enough time to grieve and the right support, we can begin to choose our next steps forward, and the words we will use to define our experiences. It is normal to feel sad or angry or to deny the reality of our situation but staying too long on this path can be unhealthy.

We encounter crossroads throughout our lives, not just at major events. We may be diagnosed with a chronic illness only once, but we revisit the implications throughout our lifetime. The information and the techniques we recommend remain valuable as we continue to deal with the defining events of our lives as the years go by.

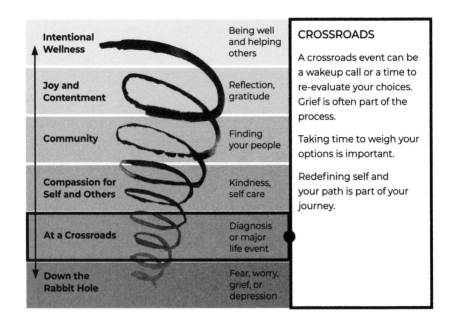

		CROSSROADS
Intentional Wellness	Being well and helping others	A crossroads event can be a wakeup call or a time to re-evaluate your choices. Grief is often part of the process.
Joy and Contentment	Reflection, gratitude	
Community	Finding your people	Taking time to weigh your options is important.
Compassion for Self and Others	Kindness, self care	Redefining self and your path is part of your journey.
At a Crossroads	Diagnosis or major life event	
Down the Rabbit Hole	Fear, worry, grief, or depression	

LIFE EVENTS

A diagnosis is a wakeup call, and for many, a defining moment in life, a time to take stock and consider options. It can provide the opportunity to reimagine what we are doing in order to change or improve.

Other life events that give a similar feeling to a diagnosis may include the death of someone important to you, a divorce, an unwanted change in employment, or a stressful move. Even though it doesn't feel like you have a voice in the matter, every crossroad provides opportunities to make choices and every person reacts differently. Even in dire circumstances, even if you are facing your last breath, you still get to choose, at the deepest, most fundamental level, how you react.

Don't be surprised if you find yourself having some major life realizations and making life-altering decisions once you have accepted your diagnosis. How and what you may change will largely define your path. We invite you to take time and care with the process. Don't rush through it. Although it can be painful, it is healthy for all of us to spend time in reflection and to grieve a loss or change of direction.

You may struggle or worry about the people surrounding you or feel that you don't have a say in how you live from day to day. You may think the time to make any changes has passed, however, it's not too late to find clarity in your own mind about what matters the most, and to find ways to honor those priorities.

For many who face the challenges of a life-changing event, it is useful to seek the help of others to help sift out and describe our emotions. A trusted friend, family member, clergy, trained counselor, or therapist can all be valuable in this process. Seeking help with the emotional aspects of life is a sign of strength and self-awareness. It is not a sign of failure or weakness. It takes internal fortitude to seek advice. It can be useful to have a place to talk and be held accountable for progress in our integration of a diagnosis or any life change.

The more we learn about wellness, the more we realize that words matter. We have not always paid attention to our word choices, or we have told ourselves that we are just talking, or that the way we say something is not important. Sometimes we have quit listening to the ways in which we tell our own stories.

Words, however, do have meaning, and studies have found that the words we choose to say lay down pathways in our brain. We have heard others share their stories, and they will say "when I got sick" referring to when they were diagnosed with Parkinson's. The word "sick" feels different from something like "when I learned I had (my diagnosis)." Though we cannot control many aspects of a diagnosis, we can control what words we use to label our experiences and how we share the information with others.

Words can change how others see us and how we see ourselves. Words define us. If we choose to describe ourselves only in the context of disease and forget about all the other aspects, we will lose the ability to be all the other things that could define us.

Speaking, sharing, and believing are powerful. The more we think wellness, the more our brain is trained to know that it is well even when we might be going through physical challenges.

The state of wellness is the antithesis of illness. It is being grateful for all that we have in our lives, and it is finding joy. It also means accepting that there are things we can no longer do and instead appreciating all the things we can do. Despite limitations, you can change your brain to find wellness and not remain focused on disease and disability.

Pause to reflect: *Think about how you describe yourself and your health. Do you pick your words carefully? Do you speak of the ways you are well and active, or do you focus on the vocabulary of illness?*

With Each Step: Nancy

In the weeks after I was diagnosed with Parkinsonism at age 58, I was reminded with each step I took. The future seemed like it had been taken out of my hands, which was a sure sign that I was at a crossroads. I changed my work to be closer to home and transferred from my children's librarian position to a less physical job as a reference librarian in a busy downtown library, which turned out to be much more demanding.

The public library is one of the last free places where we warmly greet people who come through our doors. We offer to help everyone, including some of our most down-and-out library patrons. I truly welcomed being of service and found this element of my work to be highly satisfying. I did not want to have to give up my work because of Parkinson's. The emotional grief that I experienced around this time was intense.

It took me several months before I was ready to talk about what it meant that I had a chronic illness to anyone but my closest family and friends. Even after time had passed, as I first told my coworkers, I cried. Amazingly, as I chose to share with more people, I received their easy acceptance and support. I had used valuable emotional effort to keep my diagnosis hidden, and it turned out to be a secret not worth keeping.

Today, it's uncommon for me to feel too sad or overwhelmed when I tell people that I have Parkinson's. Sometimes I even see the humor in it. There's no point in taking life too seriously when I'm trying to put on a nice touch of lipstick and my right hand has a different plan entirely. Luckily, having a chronic illness is only one aspect of who I am.

A New Name for a New Time: Kat

Early in my journey with Parkinson's, I knew that I would not be defined by a disease. I felt different once I left work and I needed to find other ways to be myself that were authentic, service oriented, and at a pace that was defined by my needs. It would be a new way of approaching my life—not defined by a goal or the needs of my family, not dictated by the tides of labor, or the timing of babies. I could not remember a time when I had ever given myself permission to be so, well, selfish. I was at a major crossroads. The time had come to take a hard look at myself and to design a life that could accommodate my hardwired need to help and contribute while also taking care of myself.

Once I started thinking about a redesign, my sense of playfulness returned. I decided the logical first step was to change my name and print a business card. Kathleen is my full name, very formal, and only used when I was in trouble as a child. My whole life I was called Kathie. All of my professional licenses listed Kathleen, but I was Kathie to the world. My parents and an aunt often called me Kat. I loved the name, but it felt too informal for my professional self. Changing my name to Kat was the beginning of claiming my authenticity. I printed up cards for "Kat Hill" with "boxer, blogger, and artist" under my name.

The process of renaming myself announced the start of a new chapter in my life. Using a title like "artist" helped me to realize that I could choose to redefine myself and follow passions in a formal way. Once again using words to take charge held power and bolstered my confidence.

I also decided to throw myself a party. The celebration was to commemorate the closure of this part of my life. I began to shift my grief into the framework that leaving my practice opened space for someone else to have their turn. It would be my turn to try something else and to celebrate and find joy.

WORKING

For some of us, our job tells the world who we are. Our work defines us, for example, "I'm a pilot," or "I own a small restaurant." For others, working is simply the means to earn money to fund our true passions, such as "I'm a bartender because it pays for my ski lift ticket." Others make just enough of a living to get by. No matter the reasons why any of us work and the way we feel about our job, working provides much of our daily structure and the financial means of support in our lives.

At some point while following a diagnosis of chronic illness, you are likely to face a change in your work status. Whether this life event is initiated by your employer, or requested by you, it will nevertheless bring you to a crossroads. This is an opportunity to review and evaluate whether you are still healthy enough to do a good job, whether your contribution is valuable and important, or if it is too demanding for you to also take care of yourself. If you are contemplating how work fits into your next phase of life, you might create a list of pros and cons and compare the different reasons for you to stay in your current job or line of work, transfer to a different job, or stop work altogether. There isn't necessarily a right answer.

Who are we if we are not working at our vocation? Work transitions are different for every person. You may want to talk to others who have changed jobs before you to help guide you. So much of our days are filled with tasks of work that it can be both troubling and exciting to imagine yourself doing something different.

Many of us can continue working for several years after a diagnosis, but each situation is unique. There isn't a formula that can predict how long you will be able to stay at your job. Whether to keep working or not depends on the type of job that you do and what your symptoms are. If your job requires a steady hand and you no longer have one, you will have to look carefully at your options. Slowness, fatigue, and tremor, to name a few typical symptoms of Parkinson's disease, can be challenging and even dangerous in the workplace.

You aren't giving up who you were in your working past, particularly if you have spent years building strong working relationships with your co-workers and proving to your superiors that you are a valuable, trustworthy employee. These qualities are not lost and may help us transition to a job that we are better suited for with new physical challenges, or retirement. As hard as it feels to tell people about a diagnosis, the trust and rapport you have will come in handy. Your co-workers may rise to the occasion and offer support and encouragement.

Regardless of your specific circumstances, it is important to learn about your benefits and to become familiar with your options. The best place to start is with your employer's Human Resources contact if there is one. You might also review your job description or contract to discover options.

Your employer may provide long term disability insurance for you, or you may have acquired a disability insurance policy in the past. There can be important requirements, and each long-term disability insurance claim is different, so you will need to read your policy carefully. Some states also offer short term disability benefits.

Social Security Disability Insurance (SSDI) is the government disability benefits program. Typically, to be eligible, you have worked in a job that contributes to Social Security and have accrued enough work credits. If you file a claim, it could take one to two years to resolve, during which time you may be drawing out of your own savings. To file a disability claim, you show medical evidence that your Parkinson's disease symptoms are severe enough to prevent you from working. Be sure you are discussing challenges with work with your doctors and that they are documenting your symptoms in your medical records. If your Parkinson's disease progresses to the point of disability, the records can help you prove your claim.

Some employers may be able to offer extended health insurance coverage to its retirees. Otherwise, if you leave your job and do not have health insurance, try to find the highest level of coverage that you can afford. If you are 65 or over, you will likely qualify for Medicare. If you are disabled but too young to qualify, you may be eligible to receive a form of Medicare. If you cannot get insurance and your income is low, you may qualify for Medicaid. Start at the Social Security Administration web page for information about any of these programs.

Telling Your Supervisor or Co-Workers

Whether or when to share your diagnosis is a personal decision, especially when choosing to confide in others where you work. Talking about your diagnosis with your manager can have real advantages. If your supervisor is aware of your condition, he or she can advocate for accommodations to help you keep working, even if your symptoms have begun to affect your performance. For example, your workplace may be able to accommodate you with a different position or work duties. You might be able to change your work schedule so that you maximize your most productive hours. Or you may need to stay home and focus on your health.

Many worry that disclosing can impact the way they are perceived. While we wish we could say otherwise, this can indeed be the case. The goal of the Americans with Disabilities Act (ADA) is to prevent workplace discrimination against those with disabilities, but it cannot control the perceptions and interpretations of others. The ADA has rules that help protect your right to keep your job and require your employer to make "reasonable accommodations." If you are concerned about being discriminated against or even fired because of your Parkinson's disease, consult with an attorney or a legal aid agency.

It is always your decision to whom you disclose details about your health but being upfront and as honest as possible is the easiest way to function. You may experience both unexpected support and tremendous relief from no longer worrying about hiding symptoms. When you talk to co-workers who are not familiar with the effects of Parkinson's disease, you will probably find that misconceptions are common and that you can play a key role in educating others. Some workplaces have employee resource groups to support and educate about accommodations, laws, and the realities of working with a disability. We encourage you to seek information and support when you are considering sharing your news.

When It's Time to Stop

For many people, the work decision is one of the weightiest topics on their mind. Should you retire? Or should you stay in the workforce? It's possible that your peak earning years, generally between the ages of 40 and 55, are no longer available to you. A chronic illness and early retirement or disability income are probably not what you were planning for.

This is a tough decision for anyone to face. Do not rush your decision and remember that every situation is different. The more research that you do and the more data you gather, the better prepared you will be.

In many cases, it will become obvious when working is no longer an option. Maybe the job requires skills that you cannot perform any more, or the demands of work will no longer be healthy to maintain. It is difficult but possible to manage a demanding career and take good care of one's body.

Parkinson's disease places a huge economic burden on our country, not the least of which are the ways it affects a person's financial well-being and ability to participate in the workforce. The total cost of Parkinson's disease to individuals, families, and the U.S. government is estimated by the Michael J Fox Foundation to be $51.9 billion annually. Of this, $25.4 billion is direct medical costs and $26.5 billion is non-medical costs like missed work, lost wages, early forced retirement, and family caregiver time (Lewis Group, 2019).

Many people that we know, when informing their managers that they have a chronic illness, have gone through a variety of different experiences. If you were performing at the top of your working abilities before your diagnosis, you could be in for a rough transition. Some have had success without needing accommodations, while others felt subtle discrimination in the workplace but were able to work through it. Maybe they don't get the plum assignments that they once did, but for the most part they can hang on and still have five to ten good working years left. Employers may encourage early transition to retirement due to performance issues. Some people were able to advocate for themselves and turned having a disability into becoming a positive role model for others. Others need to discontinue working almost immediately and find themselves quite suddenly applying for disability benefits.

No matter how much you believe that you are prepared for the day, it can still be a shock to your system to retire earlier than you had planned. One day you are in a job you like, with a flurry of people around and deadlines to meet, and the next day, you are home. It can be quiet and lonely, and there isn't any structure or urgency to your days. While you might like the freedom of managing your time and activities, you might also feel like you are drifting.

Many people find it hard to handle a job transition, at least at first. Just like a diagnosis, leaving work is a life event, which brings us back to the spiral. With any major life event, the wellness spiral is a model to understand and integrate life changes. Difficult events may take us down the rabbit hole to grieve and process. Compassion for ourselves and others, building and relying on a community, finding joy and wellness no matter your circumstance, can all be learned. We will guide you through the process in the chapters ahead. A change in employment is a major life event. Once again, movement along the spiral is not sequential or fixed, but rather a fluid process.

Pause to reflect: *If you are working now, do you have a plan to keep going? Have you made a list of pros and cons? How is working affecting your health?*

OUR AGING PARENTS AND ADULT CHILDREN

As part of the sandwich generation—those who have a parent older than 65 and are either raising a child under 18 or supporting grown children—we are asked to meet a variety of demands and it isn't always smooth sailing. Not only do we provide care and financial support to our parents and our children, but nearly four in ten say both our grown children and our parents rely on us for emotional support (Pew Research Center, 2013).

Supporting others is an overwhelming task for many people. There are options to help care for aging parents and children, but they are expensive and often not ideal, leaving few choices for many families. Assisted living, co-housing, in-law suites, and accessory dwelling units are among the many options for providing housing for aging parents who can no longer live alone. Our economic times necessitate creative ways to meet the demands of multiple generations.

The people that you consider to be your family may be biologically or legally related to you, or they might be dear friends to whom you are emotionally close. Whether you live near to each other or far away, are related by birth, marriage, or adoption, or none of these, your chosen family provides mutual support and love. For better or worse, you play significant roles in each other's lives, and never more so than when one of you has a chronic illness.

WHAT TO TELL THE KIDS

Many people with a new diagnosis are still in their child-raising years, or they have young adults at home just starting to leave the nest. Our roles shift naturally as our kids become adults, but this can become more complicated when there is chronic illness in the picture. Our job may no longer be taking daily care of our kids, but we are still helping them develop skills to fend for themselves in the world.

Kids can be torn between wanting to be independent adults and yet feeling worried about our health and the future. We aren't always sure how much to share with them regarding our changing health needs. You don't need to tell your kids any details about your health that you don't want to, or anything that your instincts caution you against. But most families can handle the truth if you present it in an authentic and caring way. Just like all the other people who love you, your kids will want to know what is going on.

We also think that kids will ask the right questions when they are ready to hear the answer. Withholding important information will not save them from feeling sad or angry or a myriad of other emotions. The best we can do is promise that we will answer them truthfully and keep them informed on important details, especially if something changes. Failing to do so may add unnecessary worry and distrust.

Sharing your experience with your growing children can be an opportunity for them to feel appreciated in a new way. The ability to be vulnerable with the ones we love most is part of the foundation of family. Being a parent is too important of a role to let it be diminished.

PROS AND CONS OF DNA TESTS

Sharing about Parkinson's disease with your kids may bring up the question about whether your illness can be inherited. In this case, your diagnosis might also become your children's diagnosis in years to come.

Like with other complex diseases, science cannot yet tell us how we came to have Parkinson's. It may be hereditary or familial, meaning it is caused by genetic factors, or idiopathic, meaning it has an unknown cause and is likely to be the result of a combination of multiple factors, both genetic and environmental. There are also theories linking micro-organisms in the gut to Parkinson's. (Li, et al, 2019).

In most cases, scientists believe that Parkinson's disease is not hereditary. Some cases are caused by genetic mutations, but again, hereditary causes of this disease are rare. Only about 15 percent of those who have Parkinson's disease have a family history (Dawson, 2021). For the rest, the cause of Parkinson's remains unknown. (National Institute on Aging, 2017).

Should you or someone in your family take a DNA test to see if they have one of the known Parkinson's genes? It is a complicated question and there is no clear answer. It is certainly easy to order a DNA testing kit online, but the results can be life-altering and the process should be considered carefully. Genetic counseling is recommended for anyone taking a genetic test to help interpret the results, whether they are expected or otherwise.

It is important to understand that genetic risk is just one piece of the bigger puzzle. Carrying a specific gene does not mean your offspring will or will not ultimately develop the disease. The same could be said about inheriting a cowlick, red hair, overbite, or dry wit.

Genetic testing is a very personal decision. Anytime that genetic testing is considered, particularly where there is no change in treatment based on any findings, experts recommend that you first discuss the impact this information might have. Be sure to consider how or if you will share results with your children. Those that share your genetics will be at risk of inheriting genetic disorders.

Once test results are seen, they cannot be unseen, so it is up to you to weigh the options. Even favorable news and reassurance may affect your family's concepts of themselves and may lead to what is called "survivor guilt" or even a sense of ostracism from the family (Quaid, 1992; Wexler, 1992).

Some people worry that such tests can create a false sense of security—or needless fear—among people who misunderstand what the results mean or who get inaccurate results to begin with. Test results may be deeply troubling, raising fundamental questions of medical vulnerability, as well as personal and social image and identity. People may perceive that they are flawed, abnormal, or may be afraid that others will see them or their children in these terms (Kessler, 1989 & Lipkin et al., 1986).

One Thousand Ways: Nancy

As the parents of a clever and resourceful young man, my husband and I quickly learned to be flexible. I took to heart a saying from the Chinese author Zhang Wei who wrote: "There are a thousand ways to live," and I soon realized there are a thousand ways to handle a parenting challenge. Our family explored a lot of options during our son's teenage years. As a result, I learned that there are plenty of right ways to be your child's best parent. We start by doing the best we know how.

Because of this mindset, Rob and I shared my Parkinson's diagnosis with our teenage son as soon as we felt calm and able. We knew our son's thoughts were preoccupied with his school and outside activities, but we also knew he has a kind and perceptive nature. We wanted to keep our lines of communication open and assure our son that we were well equipped to handle this as a family. He listened quietly and then asked questions of both of us. He wanted to know about my current health and wondered what to expect. We tried our best to answer. Our son is in college now. He continues to be clever and resourceful and sees how I incorporate what I have learned about slowing the progression of this disease.

The truth I have learned is that the future comes for our children whether we are ready for it or not. If we are lucky, our children grow up to become great adults. They make their own choices and start to build independent lives. Soon, our task becomes less about managing and more about understanding who our children have become, loving them, and respecting the way they choose to live.

Tell It Like It Is: Kat

Much like our experience with Sawyer's diabetes, Ken and I chose to share the news of my diagnosis with our children right away. I was honest that I was unsure about what the future would hold, how my diagnosis might affect my function, and that it would likely be different from that of my father.

We knew at that time and still know that we can count on each other to be honest and keep each other informed. I have pledged to honestly answer any questions that they have, even if it is hard. This approach helps them not to worry about how I am doing. They also know I will share as changes occur.

COMMERCIALISM

The world we live in moves quickly. In the information age, knowledge can be found with smartphones in an instant. The latest and greatest treatments and research are all neatly spelled out and transmitted into our hands. It can be helpful and confusing to sift through. Other people, although well meaning, will offer advice as they too seek information.

Companies that make and manufacture drugs are in the business of illness. They have a pitch to sell you a product that will treat your disease or your symptoms and make you feel better. In the case of Parkinson's disease, there are only a handful of drugs that work to combat symptoms. As a consumer, it is important that you remember that drug companies are not in the business of wellness. They profit from the treatments of our disease, and they want us to know that we are ill, because if we are ill, we want to be well. They use language that tells us we are sick, defeated and use words like "fight" to tell us what to feel and imply that they understand our symptoms. All these methods are a way to reinforce our illness and our perceived need for their product.

It is a system that is broken. Drug manufacturing and sales are big businesses in the US. The companies producing drugs also make huge profits treating what ails us. Conversely, there is not big money for drug manufacturers keeping people well.

Knowledge is powerful, but information overload is a challenge that can make decision-making difficult. We are constantly being bombarded with advertising about the newest and best, from our social media feeds to our cereal boxes. We see data and information every day. It can be hard to decipher a sales pitch from the truth. It can help to use the game "what are they trying to sell me?" with your family to tease out advertising messages. Watch commercials on TV and try to figure out what they are trying to sell. Sometimes it is hard to decipher, but it can help to get to the truth of the messaging.

As parents, we felt that it was important to teach our children how to view advertising with a critical eye. Together, we would critique drug company ads for medications and treatments. It may seem silly, but it helped our children view advertising in an informed way and to decipher what the goal of the advertising campaign was.

Over time, these messages can do more harm than good. As we discussed earlier, words matter. If we are bombarded with messages of illness, we may believe them. Surrounding yourself with healthy messages and words can have a more positive effect.

When Kat's son Sawyer was diagnosed with diabetes at the age of eight, he saw commercials about medications that all warned "if you have a compromised immune system with diabetes...." He feared death every time he was sick. In response, Kat's family changed the messaging that he heard. For every cold or stomach bug he successfully recovered from, he was told how strong he was and that his immune system was working just the way it should. His blood sugars and diabetes were treated more aggressively while he was ill, but his body was strong and kept away invading illnesses.

DIAGNOSED AT A YOUNG AGE

The average age of diagnosis for people with Parkinson's is 60 years old, but a smaller number, estimated to be ten percent of the people with Parkinson's, are diagnosed even younger than 50 years old. Those with young onset Parkinson's Disease (YOPD) have unique challenges.

It is not widely agreed upon where the age line for young onset should be drawn, because age alone does not describe their experience. Those in this stage of life may have children living at home, work at a career in peak earning years, provide support to their family, and care for aging parents. A diagnosis of chronic illness will likely have a different meaning to them than it does to an older adult who has transitioned from their career to retirement, perhaps with grown children and grandchildren. We do not suggest that it is less upsetting or difficult to receive the diagnosis if older, but the financial and social impact will vary in different stages of life. Those with young onset more frequently experience loss of employment, disruption of family life, greater perceived stigmatization, and depression (Schrag, 2003).

In our roles, we have gotten to know people with young onset Parkinson's disease in all stages of life. A remarkable Parkinson's advocate, Matt Eagles, lives in the United Kingdom and was diagnosed at age seven. He is the epitome of resilience. As an adult, he works as a disability advocate, is married with children, and recently accomplished a mid-air walk on a soaring biplane. He has had the disease for nearly 50 years. While Matt is an outlier, it is fair to say that the longevity of his disease and the impact for him is different than for someone diagnosed at age 60.

Some people believe that once you identify as young onset, you are young onset for life. We agree. The commonality of shared experience and the ability to understand the impact the disease has in different stages of life is important to many. "Young" is a state of mind and spirit. Since medicine and science have not reached a consensus with an age cut off, we don't need a cut off either.

Meet Our Friend: **Marilyn**

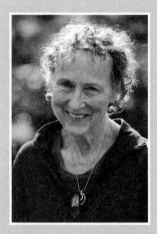

Marilyn has always loved music and dancing, and she is one of the founding members of our local Parkinson's dance troupe. She is known as a smart and loving friend to many in our community.

Marilyn was diagnosed with Parkinson's disease at age 50. A mother of four, including her youngest two, a set of twins, Marilyn continued to work for ten more years as a high school science teacher following her diagnosis. She is now in her early 70's.

Marilyn and her husband George regularly attend our support group because they, like us, were looking for an active group. They appreciate the format of the discussions and the focus on wellness. In turn, they bring a rich perspective to the rest of us about longevity and resilience. ✳

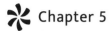

Chapter 5

COMPASSION FOR SELF AND OTHERS

"When we give ourselves compassion, we are opening our hearts in a way that can transform our lives."

—KRISTIN NEFF

BEING IN A RABBIT hole is demoralizing, and at some point, most of us decide that we are ready to climb up, dust ourselves off, and continue along our journey. In this chapter, we will show you how to move forward by focusing on taking care of ourselves with compassion and tending to our emotional and physical well-being.

Learning to be compassionate is an essential step to wellness. To be compassionate is to demonstrate a caring concern for yourself and others. We see compassion as both a state of mind and a way of taking action.

Another way to describe compassion is *being kind*. Practicing kindness to everyone, starting with yourself, is a great way to move into a life of wellness. To be kind, one is generous, helpful, thinking about other people's feelings, and also not causing harm or damage. As the Dalai Lama says, "My religion is very simple. My religion is kindness." The "small acts of kindness" and "pay it forward" movements describe ways of being in the world that are kind and compassionate toward others.

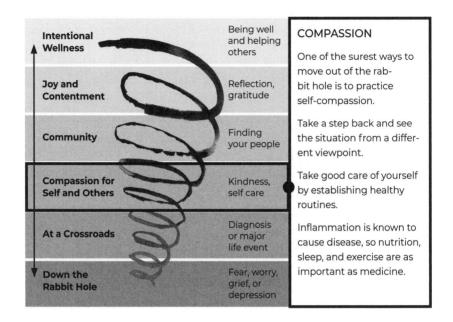

When you are overwhelmed by fear or other emotions about what the future holds, your first tasks are to ensure your thoughts are self-compassionate ones, work to acknowledge and comfort yourself, and get treatment for any emotional or physical pain you are experiencing. This is the time to start to integrate your before-diagnosis-self with how you see yourself now. For many of us, it is far easier to show others compassion than to offer it to ourselves. We hope this chapter will share some approaches to changing that.

Learning self-compassion takes intention. It requires that you pay attention to how you are feeling—peaceful, unhappy, frightened, whatever it might be—and to understand and extend compassion toward yourself. You can do this in many ways.

- Write in a journal about your actions, thoughts, and emotions, and how these are connected to the larger human experience.
- Practice mindfulness.

- Express yourself through creative outlets such as art or music, in order to create an authentic and ongoing expression of your being.

- Work through issues of grief and anxiety in therapy.

- Talk with a trusted friend.

- Exercise.

- Treat symptoms.

- Work with your care team toward your best health.

You can practice self-compassion just about any time. It is particularly useful when you recognize that you are worrying or judging yourself. The sooner you understand your own feelings and emotions, and can be honestly compassionate with others, the sooner you can live with less judgment and anxiety.

It takes introspection and thoughtfulness to be self-compassionate. Sometimes asking yourself a question about how you feel is a good way to start a dialog with yourself. Try to respond to your thoughts honestly, with love and confidence. Write yourself understanding words of comfort. Here are some examples of compassionate messages you can tell yourself:

- I am taking the best care of myself that I can.

- I am starting fresh at this moment.

- I am strong and can accomplish difficult things.

You might be someone who uses words to better understand your experience, or you might feel the most insight when talking to others. Maybe your most compassionate moments come when you are out in nature or exercising. No matter how we find it, we must have compassion for ourselves before we can practice it with others.

Research has shown that adults who have developed a secure attachment to others in life are able to build compassion more easily (Bowlby, 1990). The theory makes sense, that those who feel secure in life are able to show more compassion. We must feel good in our own skin before we can share it outwardly. A diagnosis or other major life event can shake our self-assurance and it might take some time to regain our footing. Allowing yourself the time that you need will aid in building the skill of self-compassion.

Shifting the messages that we tell ourselves from critical to kind is vital to our well-being. As we are kinder to ourselves, we have more emotional availability to show kindness and compassion to the people around us. We are more present. This principle is discussed by the Dalai Lama in *The Book of Joy* as a virtuous circle. Once one good thing starts happening, other good things happen, which cause the first thing to continue happening. As we heal our own pain, we can turn to be of assistance to others in pain. Once we are not focused on our own suffering, we are more available to help others.

Choosing your words, or the stories you tell yourself, is crucial. If the message you say when looking in the mirror is "I am fat" (all too common), that evokes an unpleasant feeling. The emotions stirred by looking in the mirror and saying "I am strong and capable" are quite different. Compassionate self-talk is the healing story we tell ourselves.

Pause to reflect: *How do you feel today? What messages are you giving yourself when you look in the mirror? Are you engaging in kind self-talk?*

TAKING CARE OF YOUR HEALTH

Your brain is the key to creating and maintaining health. If you lead with your thoughts before you take action, the rest will follow. You can be mindful and intentional about your process. What makes you feel good? What tools are the most beneficial? What changes do you want to make? What advice do you want to implement? Your choices will be specific to you. Before you change or dismiss habits, think about a plan of action and whether a change is important to you or not. Even when it feels difficult, it is within our control to think about, plan for and make changes in our thoughts and behaviors.

You have made it this far in your life by making changes and adjustments as needed. You have all that it takes to move forward and create behaviors to focus on and optimize health. You are the most important tool in your wellness arsenal.

In times of great stress, the mental toll can feel all-encompassing—and it is appropriate and normal for this to be the case. As soon as you are able to start focusing on your physical health, you can start evaluating where you are and see where you need to adjust. The factors that we describe in this chapter, specifically eating well, sleeping, and getting exercise, play a significant role in your overall wellness and even the course of the disease.

YOUR UNIQUE DIAGNOSIS

Getting an accurate diagnosis of Parkinson's disease is complicated. Currently, there is no objective test such as a blood test, brain scan or EEG, to make a definitive diagnosis. Instead, your doctor takes a medical history and performs a neurological examination. They are looking for certain physical symptoms that qualify a person's condition as Parkinson's disease.

One common diagnostic test is a medication challenge. We write more specifically about medication later, but basically, if your symptoms improve noticeably after taking the medication, it may indicate Parkinson's. If your symptoms do not improve, you likely have a different condition. We have heard people say that they were concerned when their doctor wanted them to start on medication right away, but it may have been that they misunderstood the diagnostic purpose. Be sure to ask your doctor if this is the case.

Some doctors will recommend that you have a DaTscan. This involves injecting a small amount of a radioactive drug into you and looking at it with a machine similar to an MRI. The results of a DaTscan cannot show that you have Parkinson's, but they can help your doctor confirm a diagnosis or rule out other possibilities. The scan will show how much dopamine you are producing.

It is not unusual for people with a chronic illness to get one or more diagnoses before they find the one that fits the best. Early symptoms can match other disorders, and in many cases, an accurate diagnosis is only made by eliminating other possibilities.

Some people with Parkinson's disease are first diagnosed with essential tremor, a movement disorder that causes involuntary and rhythmic shaking, especially in the hands. It can be distinguished from Parkinson's disease because it usually occurs alone, without other neurological signs or symptoms. Another diagnosis is Parkinsonism, which is a general term that refers to the group of neurological disorders that cause movement problems like those seen in Parkinson's disease, such as tremors, slow movement, and stiffness.

It is common to convince yourself that you have the wrong diagnosis or that there's nothing wrong after all. Stay curious and continue to gather knowledge about your symptoms. It may take time to find the right doctor, the right diagnosis, and the right form of treatment for you.

PRIORITIES

How we focus our lives, honor our priorities, and keep informed about treatment options is a dance we must learn. It is important to strike a balance that works for each of us individually and can be a way to show compassion and kindness to ourselves and how we view our bodies.

One of the best ways to take care of your health is to prioritize. There is an important balancing act between the time we focus on treatment versus the time we focus on living. How do we navigate the increasing appointments with different providers and therapists with all the other demands and needs for our time? Don't forget friends, family, partners, work, and hobbies, all of which are vitally important.

To get started on prioritizing, take a look at the last month or so of your calendar. For some, it may be helpful to track your time using a spreadsheet. This is a very individualized process, but sometimes counting the hours or days spent on tasks can enlighten movement or change.

Certainly, you could be 100% busy fighting disease with exercise classes, meditation, Tai Chi, physical therapy, massage and acupuncture, speech therapy, occupational therapy, neurologist appointments, and clinical trials. The list goes on. Each of these valuable adjuncts aid the mind and body, but no one has the time to do it all. It is necessary to consciously and compassionately find a way to divide your time between wellness activities and other priorities.

If all of your energy is spent only dealing with disease, you might be missing out on what is most important to you and lacking balance for the natural order of your life.

Pause to reflect: *What activities do you spend the most time on? What aspects of your life would you like to make more time for? What areas could you spread out or plan differently? How does the balance feel?*

Connections That Nurture: Kat

While maintaining social connections is important and even necessary, these connections should enhance your well-being. As I made the transition into life with Parkinson's, I received many lovely invitations from friends. I was delighted and accepted everyone, knowing that I needed to get out and stay social. I quickly learned, however, that it was time-consuming, expensive, and draining to have the same conversations over and over again.

It was confusing, having been a lifelong extrovert, that I often felt exhausted after my outings. Blessed to have many friends in my life, I was perplexed by what I perceived as a change. Was it Parkinson's?

What I came to understand is that while some relationships nurtured me, some did not. I realized that trying to cultivate too many relationships at the same time did not allow the space to grow and nurture those that mattered most. As my symptoms progressed with Parkinson's, I also found I had significantly less energy. I would need to conserve the social energy I had for those who helped to fuel me emotionally.

In my typical "planner" way, I made a list. I would make space for those on the list, meeting up, having dinner, and planning social time together. My list included some, but not all, of my family. Those not on the list, though dear to me, would be those that I would see less frequently or within the context of group settings. This process helped me to set guidelines for myself and find more intentional ways of connecting and creating space for those I love.

For those not on the list, when I was invited to an event or coffee, I would say, "I'm not available for (insert event) as I am not going out as much," or, "I have another commitment." The commitment is self-care and being less busy. Words matter, honesty is important, and I did not want to hurt any feelings. I found most people were gracious in accepting my responses and I continue these practices to this day. This practice is a way I show compassion for myself and for others in my life.

ROUTINE WELLNESS

We encourage you to continue performing all of your daily habits and regular routines for maintaining good health, even as it becomes more difficult to do some of the things that once were easy. Routines offer a way to create wellness in our lives through structure and organization. Having daily habits can greatly improve your health and be seamlessly incorporated into your life. When we are organized, it's easier to actively work toward meeting health goals. With planning, we can challenge ourselves to do such things as prepare and eat a healthy diet, and exercise consistently.

If you are looking for a way to track your health, try using your smartphone or computer to set up reminders. For example, you can set alarms to help track your meals and exercise and to remind you when to take your medicine.

In addition to maintaining healthy routines at home, it is important to visit your doctor to keep up with routine wellness checks. Make sure that your care providers have up-to-date information about your symptoms, treatments, and medications. These should include laboratory work, immunizations, blood pressure checks, and a physical examination. Your doctor may request to draw blood for several laboratory tests, including a complete blood count and a metabolic panel. These panels test your blood and can indicate any issues that exist in your kidneys, liver, blood chemistry, and immune system. Your doctor may also request diabetes and a thyroid screen. If you have an increased risk of heart attack, heart disease, or stroke, they may also request a lipid panel to check your cholesterol levels.

It is also important to care for your teeth. Regular dental checkups are recommended for everyone. Be sure to discuss with your dentist or dental hygienist any problems you are having. You might find it is harder to brush your teeth as symptoms such as tremors or rigidity can interfere with the ability to coordinate your fine motor skills. Medications can also impact the way we make and use saliva. Accommodations such as an electric toothbrush can help you maintain good habits.

Likewise, you will want to keep regular appointments with your eye doctor. Besides normal age-related problems, symptoms such as having trouble reading, double vision, and dry eyes, may be due to disease progression or medications that you take and should be talked over with a vision specialist.

INFLAMMATION

A significant part of what makes our bodies work and be well are our blood vessels. They feed all our organs. There are large and very small vessels. When they function optimally, they help all our organs work well together. When inflammation impacts our vessels, and therefore how they function, they start to break down. The smaller the vessel, the more susceptible to damage.

Most disease states are caused by an inflammatory process. When any blood vessel is inflamed, its function becomes compromised. Any dysfunction or breakdown in any blood vessel in any part of our body can lead to disease or malfunction of the organs fed by the vessels. There are simple ways to decrease the risk of inflammation in your body. The three most important are nutrition, sleep, and exercise. Sound familiar?

Can we stop or slow the inflammation? The good news is yes, it can be done. A low inflammatory diet helps. We also know that exercise decreases inflammation on a cellular level which helps our bodies prevent the process and aids in staying healthy.

NUTRITION

Just as your physical body and experience of chronic illness are unique to you, so are your nutritional needs. That's why there isn't one diet recommended for every person on the planet, nor is there one meal plan that is best for people with Parkinson's disease. Regardless, all the food that we eat plays an important role in our well-being and the state of inflammation.

Many nutritionists recommend eating a low-inflammatory Mediterranean-type diet. This diet is rich in leafy greens, vegetables, fruit, beans, and fish and is healthy for almost everyone.

A recent study also recommended the MIND diet, which combines aspects of the Mediterranean diet and the Dietary Approaches to Stop Hypertension (DASH) diet. Both the MIND and Mediterranean diet are associated with later onset of Parkinson's disease. Although the majority of food groups are similar, the MIND diet specifically encourages leafy green, berry, and poultry intake, and recommends against fried food and sweets, and to a lesser degree, milk, potatoes, and fruit (Metcalfe-Roach, 2021). Other researchers have shown that dairy products, particularly in men, may provoke disease progression, and the evidence is stronger for milk than it is for cheese or yogurt (Seidl, 2014).

Foods that cause inflammation in the body are often highly processed. Dietitians have long encouraged us to eat only ingredients that we can pronounce and foods that do not have a long list of ingredients. This is good advice for everyone and especially important if we are trying to optimize health and combat disease. We do ourselves a service by eating a healthy diet and avoiding processed ingredients. Eating organic foods that have less exposure or toxic pesticides and herbicides is also recommended. Fruits and vegetables that have edible skin are those most recommended to buy from the organic produce section.

Healthy, organic foods are often more expensive and harder to find, which can prove a barrier for many. Addressing the chasm of food scarcity globally is another topic to take on, but we acknowledge that it is a privilege to be able to find and afford organic food choices.

Most nutritional scientists believe that a diet rich in fat, cholesterol, or carbohydrates alone has only a questionable role in providing healthy nutrition. Nutrients contribute to overall health and protect cells against damage or impairment of function. A lack of good nutrition can contribute to the degeneration of our bodies, especially of neurons in the brain. The right nutrient choices clearly make a difference.

Some Parkinson's medications can exclude or require very specific foods, and even specify the amounts of protein that are to be eaten at specific times. Be sure to discuss this issue with your provider. You may also experience swallowing or chewing difficulties, in which case a functional therapist (such as an occupational or physical therapist) may be able to help you.

The science of nutrition is burgeoning. We have all heard the old adage, "you are what you eat" and the newer idea of "food as medicine." Both are strong cases for being mindful of what goes into our bodies and what we surround ourselves within our environment. Preparing food and feeding ourselves and those we love are kind and compassionate acts of daily living.

No wonder there is confusion around current diet recommendations. In the 1990s the USDA taught us about the food pyramid. At the top of the pyramid, in the use sparingly triangle, were fats and oil. We were to be eating mostly bread, cereal, rice, and pasta. All kinds of carbs.

Was the FDA wrong? It seems so. In sharp contrast to the 1990 pyramid, less than a decade later, we learned we should be eating more of the healthy fats and whole grains. White rice and pasta should be avoided and used only sparingly. White flour, white rice, white potatoes now are thought to contribute to the inflammatory processes, which translates into illness and disease.

This drastic shift in "expert" messaging has led to much confusion. When the experts don't agree or contradict their previous messaging, what does one believe? This confusion combined with our super-size mentality directly contributed to our national obesity crisis.

Consulting a dietitian can be helpful to guide optimum nutrition tailored to your specific needs. They can provide a diet plan to navigate the unique challenges you may have. Of note, most health care providers do not have extensive training about nutrition, so it is best to ask for a referral to a dietitian.

SLEEP

One of life's pleasures is to wake up well-rested and refreshed, but a night of high-quality sleep is difficult to come by for many people. If you suffer from sleep disturbances, you are not alone. Both Parkinson's disease itself and the medications used to treat it can lead to sleep problems. Many people with Parkinson's wake up frequently, are not able to get back to sleep during the night or fall asleep during the day. We can't win! We sleep when we don't want to and can't sleep when we do.

Rapid eye movement (REM) sleep disorder is also common with Parkinson's disease because it can turn off the temporary paralysis mechanism during sleep and allow people to actively act out their dream state. Many bed partners have been impacted by their partners' physical nighttime actions.

Sleep disturbances are now recognized as one of many non-motor symptoms of Parkinson's disease and have been reported in 60 to 90 percent of people with Parkinson's. Sleep disorders can impact the ability to properly function while awake and can contribute to other medical problems. Studies have shown that insomnia may be a symptom of underlying mental health issues, particularly anxiety and depression (Kay, 2018). If you suspect this is true for you, it's important to work with your provider for a treatment plan. Partnerships are hard enough to navigate, without getting into a wrestling match while simply trying to sleep.

Sleep disorders with Parkinson's are similar to those experienced by people as they age. Older people tend to wake up more often during the night and have more difficulty going back to sleep than younger people. They also tend to sleep more during daytime hours. Despite the similarities, research indicates that people with Parkinson's disease experience significantly more sleep disturbances than older people, even when adjusting for age (Gjerstad, 2007).

It can be difficult to treat a sleep disorder, so please practice self-compassion. The trick is to try to keep your stress levels low as you try different techniques for relief. This is much easier said than done, but we hope you find a useful avenue to getting sleep. To get ready for a good night's sleep, don't overlook common relaxation techniques such as rubbing your feet, sipping a warm drink, or playing quiet music.

Some other techniques that you can try are making sure that you get adequate exercise early in the day, reduce your consumption, if any, of caffeine or alcohol, especially in the evening, and reduce or avoid altogether any electronic screens such as smartphones, tablets, and television, after dinner. Be sure to talk to your health care providers so that they can partner with you and provide the support you need.

EXERCISE

"Moving slow is still moving." —Harry, a fellow person with Parkinson's

When people with Parkinson's disease say that they are fighters, they can mean it literally, and many have boxing gloves to prove it. Research has shown that exercises like boxing, running on a treadmill, biking, Tai Chi, and yoga can help in the fight against disease.

The best exercise for you is one that you will do and keep doing. Some of the best choices for exercise programs balance different aspects of fitness including strength, coordination, flexibility, and endurance. For example, studies have shown that dancing regularly has positive health benefits, both physically and psychologically. After ten weeks of attending a dancing program, people with Parkinson's in one study reported an overall reduction in total mood disturbance and a specific reduction in anger. In addition, less fatigue was found for those initially scoring higher in depression (Lewis, 2016).

Here are a few of the more unusual styles of dance that have been studied in conjunction with Parkinson's disease. All showed that dancing can increase your physical movements and quality of life.

Dancing as Exercise

- The Tango
- The Charleston
- Bollywood routine
- Cockney knees-up Mother Brown
- Saturday Night Fever

Pause to reflect: *Is there some fun or funky physical challenge you have always wanted to try? Pickleball? Clog dancing? Trampoline aerobics? Water walking? You get the idea. Maybe now is the time to try.*

For exercise to be meaningful, it should be sustained for at least 20–30 minutes at a time, at least three times a week at a minimum (Ahlskog, 2011). Experts recommend that people with Parkinson's, particularly young onset or those in the early stages, exercise with intensity as often as they can manage, for the most benefit.

Exercise has been shown to promote positive and significant effects on cognitive function, processing speed, sustained attention, and mental flexibility in people with Parkinson's disease (da Silva, et al, 2018). Don't be intimidated if you are new to exercise. Take it slowly and work with your provider. There are endless resources in print or online to experiment with moving in your own home. Joining group classes or exercising with a friend adds the benefit of being held accountable to show up.

We are not typical athletes, being women of a certain age who both have Parkinson's, but we work out at an early morning boxing boot camp that involves high intensity interval training. We run up and down stairs, jump rope, wrangle battle ropes, and punch heavy bags. We do this because we know that it may slow the progression of our disease (Dorsey, 2020), and we also do it because we have found our people at these workouts.

During the COVID-19 quarantine, our instructor sent online links to continue our workouts, knowing the importance for us to manage our disease with exercise. After being granted specific permission for her gym to remain open from the governor of Oregon, she provided an essential service with upwards of 130 people logging into workouts from around the country.

BRAIN TRAINING

Scientists have shown that our brains can literally be changed by the way we think because of neuroplasticity, the brain's ability to change and create new neural pathways. Neuroplasticity has great potential for the future as scientists learn how the brain can be retrained and repaired. The science is new, but research already shows that various forms of physical exercise lead to changes in the brain (Johansson, et al, 2020).

If our brains are pliable and can lay down new pathways over time, this provides a key to changing how we live with disease and how we learn to be more self-compassionate. The flip side is also true. If we choose to define ourselves as sick or unhealthy, we lay down that brain pathway and it becomes true.

In addition to exercise being able to change our brain, mindfully turning your thoughts into positive emotions supports coping and flourishing mental health. Upward spirals of positive emotions can counter downward spirals of negativity. Mind training interventions such as mindfulness and loving-kindness meditation are believed to be able to physically generate positive emotions that counter negative processes. (Garland, et al, 2010).

Training ourselves to think positively is possible. Rather than thinking negative thoughts, we can gently and intentionally turn our minds to thoughts of wellness. It's your choice whether you make negative thoughts your sole focus. Maybe you are already having a bad day, so you give yourself up to the fear of having a progressive brain disease. Your tremor is acting up, so you indulge in thinking about a progressive brain disease. The weather is bad, progressive brain disease. You get the idea. Your thoughts can be on autopilot, or your thoughts can turn toward being well.

Solving a Puzzle: Nancy

When I visit my dear 87-year-old mother, we often work on a jigsaw puzzle together. It's one of my favorite things to do, to sit with her and talk quietly, drink tea and catch up with each other, while we search for jigsaw pieces. Mom also solves crossword puzzles and word scrambles and challenges herself daily with an online brain game. She usually tries to match or beat her highest scores from the previous day.

Mom has lived an interesting life, growing up on army bases around the world, working as a school counselor, and being a Red Cross volunteer in New York during September 2011. When I visit, I can sometimes hear her working on her brain-training programs in the next room, fingers clicking away. Her mind is sharp, and she likes the idea that she is working to train her brain to stay healthy. It gives her a concrete plan for brain health that she can work on every day, and that alone is useful.

There has been a lot of debate about how useful brain games are for cognitive training. You can increase your game score but there isn't much evidence that the newly learned skill translates into anything usable outside of the game. The brain game mostly trains you to better play the brain game. That may be plenty of incentive in itself.

The best evidence for neuroplasticity is that it has been shown to enhance brain function when combined with physical activity. Because our boxing coach keeps up with these studies, she often likes to throw in a simple brain activity to make us think while we work out. These activities might include such tasks as answering trivia questions, counting by multiples of a given number, so 7, 14, 21 rather than 1, 2, and 3, and calling out animals, sports teams, or classic car styles alphabetically while lifting hand weights. Exercising both our bodies and minds may provide the greatest boost to our brain.

Meet Our Friend: Jeff

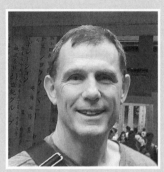

Jeff is a force and a fighter. He is always early to workouts, does the most reps with the highest intensity, and can do more pushups in three minutes than anyone we know. He is what we all strive to be in terms of fitness.

He is also a music buff. Music trivia is an integral part of our boxing workouts that helps us to exercise our brains while challenging our bodies. Jeff is a master of both. We've seen him swing and knock over a boxing dummy while sheepishly grinning as he recalls the day's rock-n-roll trivia question about a 1970s drummer.

Since Jeff's diagnosis 12 years ago, his Parkinson's has progressed. He has more times when he feels "off" and is having dyskinesia. He has recently retired from his career and has just had deep brain stimulation (DBS) surgery. Jeff is upbeat and undeterred by physical challenges. We admire him a great deal. ✳

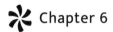 Chapter 6

COMMUNITY

"Alone, we can do so little; together, we can do so much."
—Helen Keller

A COMMUNITY CAN BE SO much more than a group of friends or a place where you live. The best communities bring together people who share common interests and relate together socially, providing friendship and companionship. In a community, you can celebrate success, share resources, and be your best self. There are powerful health benefits to being part of a community, and the connections you make can enhance and lengthen your life.

We are hardwired to live with others. From the beginning, we lived in tribes, villages, and communities. Dependence on and cooperation with each other enhanced our ability to survive. Many studies have proven that we live longer, recover better, and thrive when we are with others.

People often have several different community groups. They can be informal, for example, a relaxed group of friends who get together for a monthly card game at their neighborhood bakery, or a group can be organized and meet regularly, such as a weekly church service or a town hall.

Finding your people, where you have a deep sense of being known, being understood, and being seen, can keep loneliness at bay and will help you stay healthy. Social isolation and loneliness are well-known causes of depression, mental health problems, and physical illness, and as we acknowledged before, many of us have known the pain of feeling lonely.

If you haven't yet found a community that meets your needs, you can work to develop a new one that suits you best. Being part of a group can help you feel not so alone and can provide inspiration and motivation. Community matters, and best of all, being part of one can be rewarding and fun.

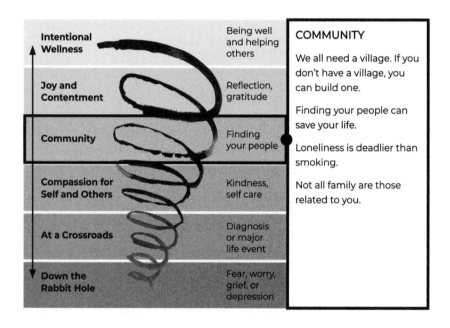

		COMMUNITY
Intentional Wellness	Being well and helping others	We all need a village. If you don't have a village, you can build one.
Joy and Contentment	Reflection, gratitude	Finding your people can save your life.
Community	Finding your people	Loneliness is deadlier than smoking.
Compassion for Self and Others	Kindness, self care	Not all family are those related to you.
At a Crossroads	Diagnosis or major life event	
Down the Rabbit Hole	Fear, worry, grief, or depression	

FAMILY AND FRIENDS

People who maintain strong family connections actually show physiological changes that enhance their well-being. Researchers have shown that our bodies release oxytocin when we have almost any form of social contact. Oxytocin is a powerful hormone that acts as a neurotransmitter in the brain. It triggers the release of serotonin (Dölen, 2013), and in a chain reaction, the serotonin then activates the reward circuitry, resulting in a happy feeling. So, having social contact contributes to happiness.

A large study was conducted with men and women recovering from heart attacks. Across the board, married people lived significantly longer than their single counterparts. The most significant factor to longevity in this study was companionship, not medication. We also know that single men die before married men. They suffer from more cancers, more heart attacks, alcoholism, and depression (Dupre & Nelson, 2019).

Friendships appear to have an even greater effect for women. Studies have measured the levels of oxytocin produced when women interact with each other. When women are feeling connected to other women, their levels are significantly higher than when alone, or even connecting with their male partners.

The psychological benefit of female friendships is strong. According to a study published in the Journal of Clinical Oncology, "women with early-stage breast cancer were four times more likely to die from cancer if they didn't have many friends. Those with a larger group of friends with early-stage breast cancer had a much better survival rate" (Samson, 2011). Part of treating our disease involves finding our people and staying connected.

Another study of women with cancer found significant positive effects from being in a support group. The women studied were undergoing treatment for metastatic breast cancer. The researchers were evaluating if women with more social support versus those with little support recovered more quickly, had cancer relapse, or lived longer. They found that those with broad social support reported better quality of life and on average lived longer than those who did not report adequate support (Kroenke et al, 2016). Being together, sharing time and experience, and having a community can improve and extend your life.

There are pockets of communities in the world called blue zones where more men and women are living past 100 years than anywhere else. Susan Pinker studied one such zone on the island of Sardinia off the coast of Italy. She found unique social factors that seemed to foster long living. The top factors derived from her many years study were that having frequent and meaningful social contacts helps us to live longer lives (Pinker, 2017). Other related blue zone research found that the happiest people in the world socialize seven hours each day (Buettner, 2011).

In blue zones, being socially integrated into one's community is a key component of long life. People in the blue zones studied are often in multi-generational living situations. Elderly family members live with children, grandchildren, and even great-grandchildren and interact with many people throughout their day. They know their neighbors and communities. They visit with people and are known by others (Pinker, 2017). Being social, connecting with people and showing up are key factors in long life in the blue zones, but also in the United States.

In the United States, many of us have moved away from the small towns we grew up in to find jobs and build lives in urban areas. In doing so, we often leave our extended families behind. We do this to "get ahead." However, if we think about how longevity is directly affected by loneliness, we should consider finding community in our new environments, especially as we age, or learn ways to stay in some of these smaller communities with our families. During the pandemic, many workers learned that they could be just as productive from remote places. Perhaps new hybrid ways of working remotely will give us more choices to live among others as we work and transition into retirement.

We can avoid isolation by spending time with others. Classes and support groups are formal ways to get involved. Informal, spontaneous coffee dates, planned weekend getaways to the beach, game nights, karaoke nights, are all ways we are connecting and thriving. Group exercise programs serve multiple benefits: meeting the need to socialize and the need to move our bodies. Though not the same as face-to-face contact, a video chat with those we care about gives us a sense of connectivity.

Those that were isolated during the recent COVID-19 pandemic and subsequent quarantine were more at risk for death than those with multiple people in small social circles. The internet's ability to bring virtual workouts into our living rooms, to provide live chats with our groups, and even to offer video text proved to be a lifeline for navigating the long months in quarantine.

Connecting and being part of a community is so important to longevity that in the United States, people are starting to rethink how, as a society, we can take better care of our aging population. We are building retirement communities that allow people to age in place while also receiving skilled care for medical issues. However, we still have a long way to go. We send our elderly to assisted living or group homes where they only interact with other elderly people when it may help people to live longer by staying integrated in multigenerational settings. We could learn a great deal about longevity from the blue zones and the ways they treat their aging seniors.

Pause to reflect: *If you do not feel like you have a supportive community, how can you find one? Are there support groups in your area, online or even by phone?*

INFORMAL GROUPS

It is hard to think of any animal for whom social behavior is not important. Humans feel the need to identify with groups, and we typically belong to many different types. People who exercise or work out together in a group tend to form tight-knit and important connections. Finding an activity you like, and finding others doing it, is a great method for tackling loneliness.

If you have children at home, you might find groups that support sports teams or the hobby interests of your kids. These groups typically meet regularly and provide for the social needs of both parents and kids. The sessions are usually informal and can happen spontaneously and voluntarily. Some last only as long as a season, and others continue on with a life of their own. Consider how long Nancy's parenting group has been together. They met at the hospital following the birth of their children. Over time, they have celebrated birthdays, empty nested, and supported each other when loved ones passed away. The parents still meet monthly. Meanwhile the babies, now adults, have refused to participate since they turned thirteen.

Likewise, Kat's friends thought they might start a book group or dinner club, since they were five mothers who worked together and enjoyed each other's company. They have been meeting regularly for the past 25 years. They found that their passion for teaching was not all they shared. They had similar backgrounds and so did their husbands. They also had children the same age. These long-term friendships are part of Kat's foundation and ones that she can rely on. And their husbands found a perfect name for the group: The Hot Mamas.

Pause to reflect: *What do you like to do? Mentor youth, race cars, restore old cameras, make art? Do you know others who enjoy these things? Can you think of a new way to meet "your" people?*

ORGANIZATIONS AND SUPPORT GROUPS

Some communities form as the result of the work of formal organizations that were created to provide services, such as not-for-profit groups, businesses, or religious organizations. One group in our local community is a non-profit that focuses on supporting clients living in Oregon and SW Washington. They provide information, education, personal support, and advocacy for a cure for those living with Parkinson's disease.

There are support groups for just about any infirmity or social need you can imagine. Members provide each other with encouragement, comfort, and advice. The groups vary in size, purpose, and scope, but regardless of the group joined, participants are assured of a confidential and safe environment where they can receive support and help others. We started our own support group when neither of us could find a group like us.

We wanted to build a group whose focus was on living well and managing Parkinson's disease. We decided to host a happy hour group. Since its inception, our group has a mailing list of over 75 people. We meet monthly and have a core group of a dozen or so. The not-so-regular members pop in and out as their schedules allow.

Once we started to talk about our ideas for a support community, other people began giving us ideas and names of people who might be interested in joining us. We worked with our local organization, Parkinson's Resources of Oregon, to form our young onset support group. We chose to launch our initial meet up at a local tea house and eventually moved to a pub.

Although we call ourselves a young onset group, we have members who are not young in years. They were looking for a group with a positive focus. All are welcome. Partners, spouses, and friends are all invited to join us. We have hosted speakers that talk about acupuncture, working with Parkinson's disease, accommodations we might ask for at work, and we have discussions about hobbies and travel. The focus of the group is on health, and we enjoy sharing a meal and a pint. We don't wear name tags. We are a group of people hanging out who all have a diagnosis in common, focusing on living, not disease. We are a community.

In our roles as support group facilitators, we meet people who are newly diagnosed, and it isn't unusual for one or all of us to laugh or cry together or both. That's one of the strengths of having a support group. Although there are days when having Parkinson's disease can feel like such a loss, we've all been through it and can help each other through the hard times.

The care partners involved in our group started a support meeting on their own. Most of the group are men. Kat's husband, Ken, sets a meetup time and place designed to meet and discuss the unique role of being a care partner or caregiver. The focus for the first half of the meetup is an event of some sort- art museum, exhibit, hike, etc. They wander around the site or take a hike, then they venture to a coffee shop to talk. Their format is informal and atypical for a support group. It appeals to the members for just this reason.

Both our young onset and care partner support groups strive to take members where they are and we work to direct, or re-direct conversations towards positive, solution-focused discussions. We have found that people are attracted to the positive tones of the groups and recognize the benefit of having community support.

Sometimes an exercise group can lead to a meaningful informal support group. A highlight of the week for us is our Saturday workouts just for women with Parkinson's disease. The workouts are tough and fun. The best part about working out is when we are done, it is time for coffee and catching up. All of us get excited to share the week's news, often talking over one another. We have nurtured each other through marital strife, surgeries, hospitalizations, drug complications, and injuries. We take time to listen, to see with a deep level of understanding because we are all co-existing with the same disease, facing many of the same challenges. We laugh, cry, giggle, share, and love one another. The Saturday boot camp and coffee club meets our needs for our physical and social health.

Finding My People: Kat

I sought out a Parkinson's disease-specific exercise program and support groups before I had a formal diagnosis. This was not just because I had read that these things slowed the progression of the disease, but because I needed to find a community that understood what was going on in my body and my mind. I felt alone in my journey and my experience having teenagers at home, caring for aging parents, and having new symptoms that halted my career. Once the diagnosis was made, I was even more certain that I needed others to help me navigate the unknown.

Many support groups had great attendance, but no one was like me. Most of the attendees were much older than me, retired, and discussed medications and issues related to retirement. I hoped to find discussions of wellness, when to start medication, how to manage work and teens, how to plan for the financial burden of leaving work earlier than planned, how to find hope as a woman in her fourth decade with a long life ahead.

My husband, and I attended several groups together and found the groups all similar in makeup, until I found a support group that was scheduled to meet at a local hospital on a Saturday morning. We arrived and found a dark conference room and only one other person—Nancy. It was soon evident that the group was not meeting. However, with trepidation, we decided to stay and share our stories with each other.

Sharing the Experience: Nancy

Early on in my diagnosis, I had a lot of questions and no one to ask for support. I was looking for people like myself who would understand what I was going through. I wanted to find kindred Parkinson's friends who were in a situation similar to mine, in that I was working full time and had a young teenager at home to raise.

When Kat and I met at that first support group, we quickly realized how much we have in common. Between us, we hold degrees in public health, journalism, nursing, midwifery, and library science. We were women with Parkinson's disease at midlife. That day, we found our community in each other, and a friendship was born that is a lifeline for us both.

We found each other because we had to. We both had been anxiously seeking others who wanted to share the experiences of living with Parkinson's disease without surrendering other parts of their lives. We shared our stories of diagnosis and how alone we were feeling. This meeting planted the idea of building our own support community.

CARE PARTNERS

Your care partner is someone that you have chosen specifically for their support and encouragement, whether it is your spouse or partner, a relative such as a parent or sibling, a close friend, or someone else within the circle of people that you know and trust. Some people do not have an automatic or obvious care partner. For those, we recommend seeking out local organizations who can help you to build your team early in your journey. Many have social workers who will know where to seek support.

People sometimes use the terms "care partner" and "caregiver" interchangeably but they are distinctly different roles. A care partner provides support to you while you still manage your condition independently. A caregiver, paid or unpaid, helps you with activities of daily living such as eating, bathing, or going to the bathroom. With a care partner, there is often a mutual sense of purpose because each person in the partnership has a role in the care and support provided.

Your needs and physical requirements may change as your illness progresses, and so may your relationship with your care partner. It's important that you feel comfortable together and are committed to open communication as needs change. Being a care partner can come with a lot of responsibility and unique forms of stress.

Frequent communication is imperative to working with your care partner. It includes talking about the good, the bad and the ugly. It is not complaining to ask for help or to accurately describe a new symptom or if an intervention is not working.

It is important to thank your partner often for their help, input, and care. For care partners, if a symptom is hidden or ignored, it can feel like they are being shut out and left to guess about what is happening for their partner. It is a crucial part of communication to discuss boundaries. Both the person with Parkinson's and the care partner or caregiver needs to be honest about what tasks they are comfortable with and those they are not.

It can be helpful to set times to check in with your care partner about how you are doing, just like you would your physical therapist or your doctor. This sets the expectation that you will be discussing what is going on, gives both parties a chance to collect and organize thoughts around the topic, and honors everyone's time. It saves the person with Parkinson's from feeling like they are complaining and allows the care partner space and a mindset to listen. Everyone needs encouragement and the freedom to share their perspective on how they feel. Are they noticing any new behaviors, positive or negative? Any change in symptoms they may be concerned about? All involved should be allowed to share the positive and negative in a safe way. In a care partnership, both parties give and receive something of value.

From Provider to Patient: Kat

Accepting help can be a humbling experience. Trouble with my hands, change in gait and balance are at times a challenge for me. Multitasking is no longer a skill I can count on. These combined "new normals" make it challenging to accomplish many simple tasks.

There is a grace, however, in learning to accept help. I try to remember caring for my mum as she battled cancer. I knew she was proud and independent. She and I maneuvered well together, and she asked for my assistance when needed while I tried not to hover. I am trying to learn to ask for help before I am frustrated and to accept help that is offered sooner.

Aging and infirmity are a nearly universal human experience. I am grateful that I have lived as long as I have, not everyone gets this privilege. How we live, how we learn to navigate the hard and humbling aspects of illness and aging will define our character. Learning to accept that we all need help sometimes and that perhaps it is simply our turn to receive it may help us keep perspective.

I have spent a better part of my own life caring and giving to others. Though it can be unnerving and uncomfortable, I am trying to learn grace in letting others help me. Keeping in mind how good it can feel to be of service to others reminds me that the cycle of life, of caregiving is going full circle.

Hearing the diagnosis of Parkinson's disease as a health care provider meant I already knew about progression and the eventual end game. During my training, I cared for patients in a Veterans Administration hospital on a neurological unit who were suffering from Parkinson's, Alzheimer's, and other neurologic diseases. I watched and provided care as their neurologic system failed them. I also have watched how Parkinson's affected my father and two uncles. I witnessed my strong, proud father slowly lose control over his balance, cognition, movement, and memory with vascular dementia from the disease.

For me, there had been nowhere to hide from the facts, no gradual easing into what Parkinson's is, no slow bits of knowledge to bite off, process and integrate. Just the cold hard fact that I have an incurable progressive degenerative brain disease.

The transition from providing care to patients and my aging parents to receiving care was a profoundly humbling process. Due to my career, I was trained in the nuances of performing physical exams—how to methodically listen to heart and lungs, how to test cranial nerve function, how to perform a pelvic exam, how to document normal and abnormal findings. I was proud of my skills and practice; I had a light touch and clear communication with my diverse patient population. I communicated in a straightforward manner and always kept in the front of my mind that touching a patient's body, sharing intimate space, and helping them give birth was an honor. Patients are vulnerable and allowing me, even paying me, to share the intimate space of a birth was nothing short of a privilege. Being vulnerable is uncomfortable and scary. These aspects were the art of my practice.

When the tables turned and I was the patient, I was no different. I was scared and vulnerable. What was different was that not all providers share my approach to caring for patients. I expected the same level of care that I practiced and was disappointed when some fell short. For many clinicians, their knowledge base was strong, but I found the art lacking. I was often disheartened after an office visit. I had high expectations of being able to communicate while also feeling cared for. Were my standards unrealistic? Could I find someone who shared my values and whom I could partner with?

Being a patient is a dehumanizing experience for many of us. Answering the cadre of intimate health history questions. Being assessed (looked at head to toe) for what your body can and cannot do under the watchful eyes of another human being while wearing little clothing is humbling at best. During this exam all the data is noted, written down, ranked, and scored by the practitioner performing the assessment. I understand what they are looking for and why. It is, however, an awful feeling to not be able to will my body to perform the tasks I know they are looking for. I know the "answers" to the test but can't make my body deliver. Tap your foot, bring your fingertip to mine then to your nose. "Can you do it faster?" they ask. I wish I could.

At times, I could not even open the bottles holding my medication. What kind of cruel joke is that? Yes, we know you have a movement disorder and have trouble using your fingers. To treat this, we are going to give you tiny pills in a bottle that takes great manual dexterity to open. Or perhaps the medicines to help you are in a single dose, vacuum sealed container that requires you to push out individual pills. Could this be more challenging? Oh, and we would like you to take those tiny pills and slice them in half. You'll need a pill splitter, not a problem. It really is a comedy of errors, especially if my medicine is wearing off. One could laugh or cry at the absurdity. I try mostly to laugh it off. Medications are childproof and patient proof!

I wish I had some special insider knowledge to share. The reality is that I am navigating the process as best I can, and it is a new role for me. I will share, however, that it is absolutely your right as a consumer of healthcare to choose providers that you trust. If you do not care for someone's bedside manner or if you are uncomfortable, say so. If your needs are not being met, say so. You are paying for a service. Do not settle for poor service, this is your health. You have too much at stake to work with those you do not feel comfortable with.

Meet Our Friend: **Kim**

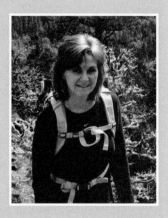

Smiling and strong, Kim shows up to boxing class. Even with a broken elbow, she comes. She may sit and cheer us on. Or walk on the treadmill at a slow pace, but she is there. We have learned to pay attention in case she has brought home-baked treats, because Kim can cook. We need our fellow Parkinson's boxer and fighter, and she needs us, her friends.

For over a dozen years, Kim bicycled ten miles to work. She was an administrative assistant when she was diagnosed at 49 years old. Her symptoms and medications made her sleepy, and she spent her breaks taking short, necessary naps. As the sleepiness got worse, she found herself nodding off during her workday. Her employer noticed and actively encouraged her to retire early. Kim wanted to keep working but didn't feel like she had the option. For her, there wasn't a celebration or the rite of passage that comes with many retirements.

No longer working, Kim expresses her creativity by connecting with her friends, designing one-of-a-kind beaded jewelry, and baking treats for her community. ✳

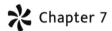 Chapter 7

JOY AND CONTENTMENT

"The most beautiful people I've known are those who have known trials, have known struggles, have known loss, and have found their way out of the depths."

—ELIZABETH KUBLER-ROSS

A JOYFUL LIFE PRODUCES POSITIVE energy and encourages us to live the best we can today. It is a life filled with gratitude and a willingness to be of service to others. The path to finding joy lies in channeling our thoughts and actions. Everything that we do and think and say determines how happy we are. It has nothing to do with what's outside us, but everything to do with how our brain works. Joy is, quite literally, within us.

In this chapter, we describe the steps to finding joy and contentment using our spiral. We want to convey that an integral part of the process is acceptance that low times will occur. Moments will be spent with thoughts in the rabbit hole, and grief with new symptoms or loss will occur. This is an all but inevitable part of living with a chronic disease. When low times exist, you know you can return to joy because you have laid the groundwork to do so.

When we shift our focus away from chronic illness and toward wellness, our perspective changes and we begin to make choices that help us thrive. It is a positive mindset that we can adopt no matter the circumstance that life presents. We lay down neural pathways that make joy our habit, and it becomes the default, not the exception.

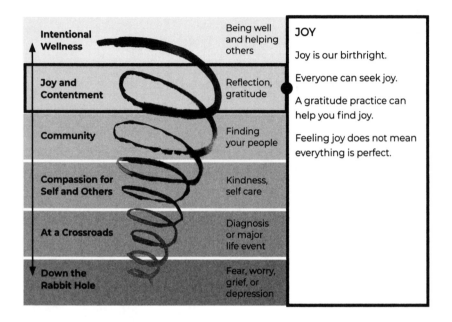

REFLECTION

The more we practice creating and experiencing joy, the more joy we find. It's a simple premise but one that requires intention, thought, and mindfulness. Intention can be as simple as a plan to look for and find small moments of joy in your day. Take a moment to notice what you feel in your body when you acknowledge a joyful experience. Be present in a moment of joy.

Do we deserve joy? Unequivocally, unabashedly, resoundingly yes! We understand this concept is difficult for many to embrace. Deserving joy feels self-centered and egocentric. It sounds juvenile. Isn't happiness enough? For some people it is, but we have found that the more we practice thinking about joy and compassion, the more cemented these impulses become and our older, critical, and un-joyful pathways fade away.

For our dear friend Karen who lost her teenage daughter to suicide, it's been more than ten years, but her grief is still fresh.

"You have to be careful about using the word joy," she told us. "It's too much."

"It's a lot," we agree. "And we're worth it."

We are not saying it's easy to learn that we deserve joy. However, don't you think, after all her suffering, Karen deserves to feel joy? Now we know that the more she practices joy, the more she will find it. Even if she only chooses it in the smallest of moments, it will get easier over time to be joyful.

In the *Book of Joy: Lasting Happiness in a Changing World*, the Dalai Lama and Archbishop Desmond Tutu discuss the benefits and challenges of living a joyful life. Despite their hardships—or, as they would say, because of them—they are two of the most joyful people on the planet.

When asked "Do you wake up with joy?" the Dalai Lama answered, "If you develop a strong sense of concern for the well-being of all sentient beings and in particular all human beings, this will make you happy in the morning, even before coffee."

Archbishop Tutu later added, "Our greatest joy is when we seek to do good to others."

If we are not focused on our own suffering, we are then free and open to aid others. When we find joy, we can in turn, help others, and so the cycle continues and grows. It is a practice that can have a great impact on our world.

Guaranteed to bring joy, a list:

- Flamingos moving in unison
- Ice cream cone
- Infant's smile
- Belly laugh

- Hot chocolate
- Warm bear hug
- Singing at the top of your lungs
- Sandy feet
- Watching a movie with friends
- Whoopie cushion

- Pot of homemade soup
- Farmer's market
- Warm pie
- A dress with sparkles
- First class upgrade
- Books
- Hand knit mittens
- Dancing with friends

Sometimes we all need to pause in our busy lives to rest, re-assess or re-evaluate. It is easy to get so caught up that we don't take a few moments to check in on ourselves.

Without knowing what he was doing, a young boy, when giving himself his insulin injections instead of thinking about pain, thought of flowers and daisies. This allowed his brain to learn to associate something positive instead of something dreadful with the necessary injection. Scientists have found that if we practice seeking joy and being joyful, it trains our brains to find joy more easily. We now know it is possible to train our brains to be happy (Dahl, 2020).

Stephen Hawking is a remarkable model for living with an incurable brain disease. He was diagnosed with Amyotrophic Lateral Sclerosis (ALS), a lethal neurological movement disorder with a poor prognosis and short life expectancy, and he went on to publish several books. He did not let his diagnosis or physical challenges allow him to stop writing, speaking, thinking, creating, and loving. He spent a great deal of time pursuing his abilities instead of focusing on his disability. As a result, we can speculate that this helped him to live substantially longer than many others with ALS.

What is on your list? *Jot your ideas down and keep them handy so it is simple to pull out and read through when you feel at a loss for finding joy. Add to it over time when you find moments in which you find yourself delighted.*

GRATITUDE

Living a life filled with gratitude is a practice, an intention, and a way of being. For some, it is part of a spiritual practice in which prayer and contemplation call for reflecting on gratitude. For others, it is a way to remember the aspects of our days for which we are most thankful.

You can start practicing gratitude at any time. There is no special technique to learn and no serious time investment. All that you need to do is reflect on what you are grateful for. Many people have incorporated writing about things they are grateful for in gratitude journals. Instead of, or in addition to, journaling, you can thank people, in person or in writing.

Many people maintain a gratitude practice. By making a formal written process, it can prompt more thought about it during each day and help document the practice. As you take time each day to start reflecting, even for a few moments, it can become a habit.

Much research has documented what happens to our brains when we practice gratitude. Certain parts of the brain are stimulated and produce the neurotransmitters, dopamine and serotonin. These make us feel good, much like the reward centers in our brains that are stimulated when making art. We all want to feel good as much as we can and adding a practice is one way you can try.

An established gratitude practice helps on difficult days when we question our abilities, and our minds play games with us. If we start to doubt that we can accomplish a task or that we deserve to live a peaceful, contented life, we can choose despair, or we can choose to be grateful.

Living with a chronic illness doesn't mean that we can't still accomplish many of our goals.

It can be all too easy to focus on our losses, especially when we live with loss every day. If we can no longer work, we find ourselves mourning the loss of our daily routine. The same is true if we are continuing at our jobs. It takes courage to be an ambassador for those of us working with a chronic illness. We are performing our own version of community service just by showing up. Even if we are symptomatic from a progressive disease, we are still here, smiling and caring for each other on our individual paths. We all have so much to give.

It doesn't so much matter if something good is on the horizon, but that we make it so. Feeling gratitude can be as simple as being thankful for different moments of the day. We can appreciate such things as seeing friends at an exercise class, setting out clothes for the day, gathering ingredients for a shared meal, or even just making a list with some enjoyable tasks to complete.

JOURNALING

We have filled numerous journals with words, pictures, and notes about our journeys. Do you have a journaling practice? Many are intimidated by the idea that a journal, or diary, must be filled with complete sentences and coherent thoughts. However, there is evidence that writing things down and journal keeping can improve well-being. Journaling has been linked to creativity, spiritual awareness, and expansion of self. Studies also note that participants identify and work through feelings, improve relationships and gain insight into themselves when journaling (Stuckey and Nobel, 2019).

In her book, *Syllabus: Notes from an Accidental Professor*, Lynda Barry details a process she assigned to her college art students. She required that they purchase a composition notebook and made time daily to create a page. Each page would include a section of what that student did, saw and heard. The fourth section was for a quick sketch of what they saw that day (Barry, 2014).

Her method was written about by a New York Times author who noted "In Barry's class, every writing exercise is a repeated ritual. At the beginning of each one … students slowly draw a spiral on a sheet of paper. Barry (then) recited a poem. It's the same poem every time, by Rumi, and Barry recited it quickly, her head down, her fingers tented before her. "You're in your body like a plant is solid in the ground,' she intoned, 'yet you're wind." (Kois, 2011)

This suggested format makes it easy to jot down thoughts. For many, this relieves the pressure of feeling like all thoughts must be beautifully composed. Barry encourages "playing" in the journal. If you keep a regular practice, it will take no time to fill up your notebook. As you develop your practice, you may find you want to use a different medium. There are so many options available. If you like adding watercolor, or paint, you may consider a heavier paper that does not buckle with wet media added.

We encourage you to add a fifth element to the format—gratitude. Each day, add a short list of things you are grateful for. Even on the toughest days you may find gratitude in things you have not ever considered, maybe for electricity or flushing toilets or curbside garbage service.

Below are a few examples of journal pages following Barry's format with the addition of the gratitude section. These are done using the standard composition notebook and notes of gratitude added diagonally or as part of the text.

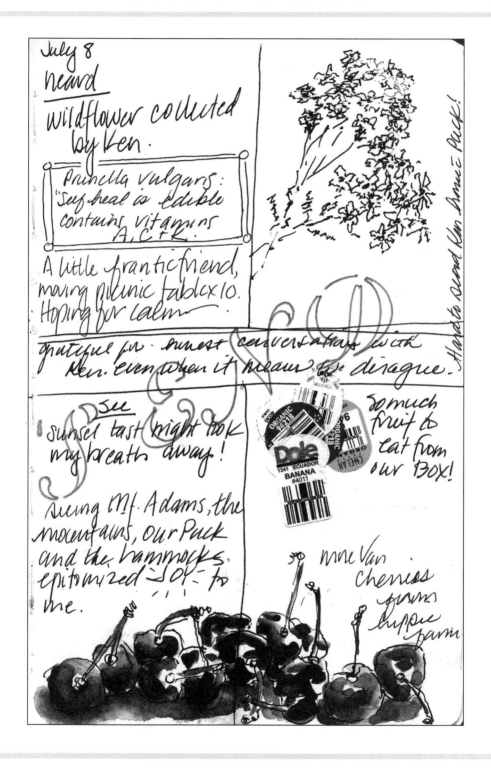

July 8
heard
wildflower collected
by Ken.

Prunella vulgaris:
"self-heal" is edible
contains vitamins
A, C, + K.

A little frantic friend,
moving picnic tables x 10.
Hoping for calm.

grateful for honest conversations with
Ken. even when it means we disagree.

Hard to read Ken Annie Puck!

see
sunset last night took
my breath away!

So much
fruit to
eat from
our Box!

seeing Mt. Adams, the
mountains, our Puck
and the hammocks.
epitomized JOY to
me.

more Van
cherries
from
hippie
farm

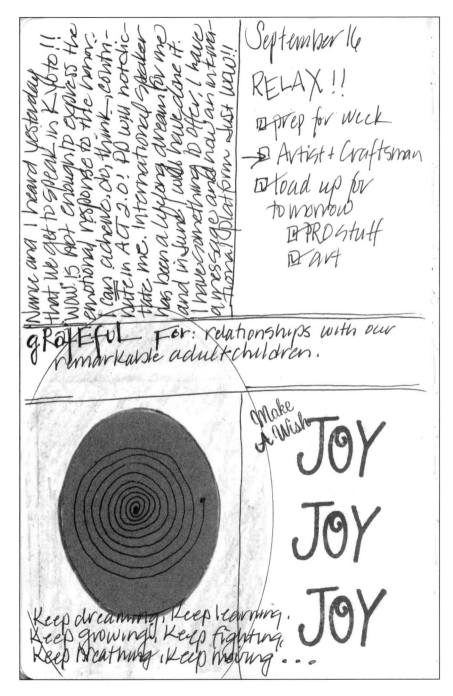

Kat's journal pages based on Lynda Barry's Syllabus *book*

CREATIVITY

Learning a new skill or taking on a hobby can help to enrich your health. You may find new skills that deserve exploration, new roles to learn about, and new horizons to see. Focusing solely on your own well-being is not enough for well-rounded health. The focus of life and health must be broad and balanced because we are complex and multi-faceted beings. We go to work, recreate, exercise, consume, eat, have relationships, family, and the list goes on.

There is evidence that people may become more creative after a diagnosis, or even develop a new interest in creative pursuits (Inzelberg, 2013). Artistic creativity may emerge in people as a result of being treated with levodopa and dopamine agonists. It's not clear exactly why levodopa treatment leads to creative awakenings in some people, but their creative expressions are often reported as being very beneficial.

Any sort of creativity—writing, visual art, music, or dance—has been shown to have positive effects on health for everyone. Developing a personal creative habit, when healthy or ill, has proven benefits. Studies have found that hospital stays can be reduced when patients take part in visual and performing arts interventions during their stays (Stuckey and Nobel, 2019).

The power of creating and experiencing music cannot be denied. There have been several studies that show that drumming improves the symptoms of Parkinson's. It boosts the immune system, activates the brain, and releases endorphins. It's a great reason to gather with other people, to share in a common experience, and to make such joyful noise.

There are lots of artists around the country who are experiencing the power of creativity. For example, Kelly Rae Roberts is an artist from Oregon. She was a medical social worker before becoming a successful mixed media artist, author, and teacher. She believes and teaches that being creative can be a way to heal and find joy. Creativity, music, painting and making art can be a way to express and find joy and wellness. You can read more about her at www.kellyraeroberts.com.

Getting Creative: Kat

Many say that learning to paint with watercolor is an exercise in letting go. Observing and studying objects and scenes to sketch and paint involves patience. Making art in a sketchbook helped me learn to transition from a highly scheduled life to one with stillness and observance.

I started painting as I was seeking a diagnosis. In a time that I was feeling little control in my life, learning to let go of flowing watercolor pigment was an exercise in faith and surrender that directly translated to what was happening with my body and my life.

Gathering all the supplies, learning to mix colors, and needing to relax and observe contributed to my enjoyment of the process. In order to paint something, you must study it. In order to study, one must be still and focused. Under the guidance of an experienced artist and teacher, I learned to focus my thoughts before tackling a sketch or painting, calming my mind, and my inner critic, with deep slow breaths. My shower practice paved the way for me to learn to do this in other places.

I quickly adopted the phrase while trying to paint, "It is the process, not the product, that matters." I do not aspire to become a famous painter. I want only to be in the moment and produce something of some likeness to the object at hand. I create my interpretation of what I see but not a replica. This mentality served me well with my process of learning to paint and of navigating a new and complex disease.

Be in the moment, observe and trust the process, accept what is.

The still activity also serves me well when I need to slow down my pace or take a rest. I need to do this more often as my symptoms progress. When we travel, I may choose to stay put at a location and sketch while my family explores more on foot. This allows us all to feel good about our experiences. I do not feel like I hold them back and they know I love my painting and sketching practice. It has been a most welcome adaptation.

Making art stimulates the reward centers in the brain and can enhance production of dopamine, which further enhances feelings of well-being. Because people with Parkinson's do not make normal amounts of dopamine, any added source is most welcome.

A New Freedom: Nancy

I have heard stories of people who suddenly discovered they were painters, sculptors, or creative writers at heart, but I didn't expect to be one of them. My urge to be creative is connected to my interest in birding, and I enjoy painting images of birds. So far, my hands are steady enough to wield a paintbrush, and I have spent lots of lazy afternoons sketching the variety of birds that I see in our backyard and then adding vivid watercolor paints. For the holidays, I painted original bird cards to send to friends. Because I have never considered myself to be an artist before now, I feel an enormous freedom to create whatever I want.

I was initially inspired by Kat's watercolor and multi-media artwork, and I began to read about color theory so that I could mix vibrant colors from different tubes of paint. I would never have guessed that combining equal parts of aquamarine blue and burnt umber would make a lovely smoky gray tone. I've found lots of tutorials and ideas for beginning painters online and I've checked out several books for beginning painters from our local library. It pays to be a librarian when you know how to locate resources.

Pause to reflect: *What creative endeavors call to you? What new expression are you interested in learning more about? Are there others that inspire you?*

LAUGHING

Little seems as immediate and warming as a full, long, laugh. It is a physical and emotive act that lightens even the heaviest of burdens. It releases endorphins and literally changes our physiology, just like we hope our medicine does. In a nutshell, it is powerful. It is medicine. It is soothing and healing. We all know how to do it.

How do we do more of it, get more of it, prescribe more of it? We first must invite more into our lives. Sometimes just living life will put you into situations that spark laughter. Trying on bathing suits with a movement disorder is a set up for either a good laugh, or cry, or both.

Consciously choosing that we want to laugh more is an invitation to find more to laugh at. Choosing stories that bring laughter, or movies that tickle your funny bone over somber, weighty tales, can add levity to your world. When finding methods of distraction or entertainment, it can be powerful to find light or funny things. There are endless comedies that can be streamed to your smartphone, laptop, or television.

There are experts that specialize in laughter and fun, even in the face of illness. Medical clowns employed in children's hospitals are such experts. Research has shown that children attended to by medical clowns during procedures on the medical oncology unit report as much relief with clowns as with a strong sedative (Rimon, et al, 2016). If children can experience comfort and relief with laughter and the antics of a bedside clown, then surely, we all could benefit from a good chuckle.

We have experienced much hilarity since our diagnosis. Sometimes, we laugh at ourselves stuck in dressing rooms, other times we can laugh with and for one another.

On the Funny Side: Nancy

Just about everyone I know that has Parkinson's also has a great sense of humor. When Kat and I get together, we might start out serious, but it isn't long before we crack each other up. We start talking about something that happened to us. You can see our crinkly eyes when we start to giggle (wait a minute, crinkly? Does that mean wrinkly?), and before you know it, tears are rolling down our cheeks.

Kat and I like hanging out with our Happy Hour support group friends. I remember the night we all ordered a pizza to share, and when it came, there was a nice pizza and a pizza cutter. But the pizza wasn't cut! Now, I ask, who can cut a pizza at a Parkinson's party? It sounds like some tangled tongue twister! It's not like we had a bunch of steady hands there. But it was great to be able to laugh about shaking with people who get it and are okay with a crooked slice of pizza.

The same Happy Hour support group has a white elephant exchange every year over the holidays and I tell you, people with Parkinson's have the strangest ideas about what makes a good white elephant gift. If you have ever participated in one, you know that there actually are no good gifts, just funny ones. One year, there was a wrapped pair of wooden children's shoes that big Bill picked. They didn't quite fit him, by half. Then Kat told us about bringing a wrapped speculum to an exchange with her midwife friends, which made every woman there who had ever had a Pap smear, laugh. Someone else told a story about once unwrapping a gift of a slightly used Squatty Potty. Hey, wow, thanks, I think.

The perennial favorite that we keep our eye out for every year is the book featuring prom photos from decades past. Lots of pastel Gunne Sax floor-length formals and big feathered hair and gaudy wrist corsages. No, that isn't me in that lovely apricot sleeveless dress with a turtleneck, and that definitely isn't my date with the flared bell-bottom tux pants and cowboy boots. Although who doesn't admire those fashion-forward, big frilly looks.

The Smile Bus: Kat

I always share with my children that no one knows if Parkinson's will ultimately "get" me. Life is full of risks and obstacles. Spending life fearing death feels like an act of futility. We will all die one day. None of us knows what the cause of our demise will ultimately be. I like to say, yes, I have Parkinson's but ultimately, I have little control over the "what" that causes my death. My son always says, "Mom, don't stand too close to the buses." Sage advice I should have taken in Japan.

Several of us were out touring gardens and shrines. There were many other tourists navigating a particularly busy parking lot. In Japan, they drive on the opposite side of the street than I am used to, and I failed to remember this and looked the wrong way. There was quite a bit of confusion and traffic as I stepped out onto the road and was quickly pulled back onto the sidewalk by friends narrowly missing being hit by an enormous tour bus. The most ironic piece of the story was the name on the side of the bus "Smile Tours." My friends and I shared a good laugh after the bus went by. If one is to be hit by a bus, better it be a happy one.

Meet Kat's Father: **Dr. Ray R Scott**

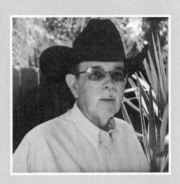

Once a small-town mayor and general dentist, Kat's father was best known for his cattle roping. He had a thriving private general dentistry practice in a small town in the central valley of California. He was also an expert in Wild West history and taught a course at the community college titled "Outlaws of the Wild West."

Most comfortable in boots and a saddle, he retired from his practice at the age of 70. After his retirement he hired himself out as a ranch hand. He wrangled cattle, tended, and mended miles of fence and built a gate that bears his name, "Ray's Gate." He spent down time at home sewing leather saddles with a parachute harness sewing machine. He crafted pieces that were works of art with his plethora of hand tools made for leather (and some for teeth!).

As the years passed, he started to notice rigidity and balance challenges. At the age of 76, he was diagnosed with Parkinson's disease. He stopped riding horses and he and his wife moved to be nearer to her family. He stayed active sitting on a rodeo board of directors, walking and having coffee with "his cronies," and participated in a research study that chronicled the possible correlation of crop dusting and Parkinson's disease. The results of that study would be presented some years later at the World Parkinson Congress in Portland, Oregon, the year Kat was diagnosed.

As the disease progressed, he lost his hand dexterity and the ability to leatherwork. After living with Parkinson's disease for 7 years, he suffered several challenging falls and qualified for hospice care. He lost his battle with Parkinson's disease at the age of 83. He passed away peacefully in his sleep at home in 2017. ✳

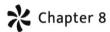 Chapter 8

INTENTIONAL WELLNESS

"Once we believe in ourselves, we can risk curiosity, wonder, spontaneous delight, or any experience that reveals the human spirit."

—E E CUMMINGS

MANY OF US LEARN to live in a way that focuses on our overall well-being. We believe that it is possible to do this while at the same time accepting the reality of having a chronic illness. We have found a personal place of balance and intention among all the wellness components that have been described in this book so far.

Intentional wellness is time spent taking care of yourself, enjoying a vibrant, supportive community, and helping others to thrive. When you act with intention, you focus on what you can do and not on the dysfunctional, broken, or ailing parts. It means taking the best care of your health, while recognizing and steering away from emotional states that do not serve you. By doing so, you can make the most of the time you have, feeling well and joyful.

There is not one widely accepted understanding of what it means to act with intention. It may be one thing for one person and hold a subtle difference to another. Here are some ways of defining intention:

"Being wholeheartedly engaged in what you are doing and what is going on, right here, right now, physically, mentally and emotionally."

"Taking responsibility for yourself and your life."

"Having a purpose behind your actions."

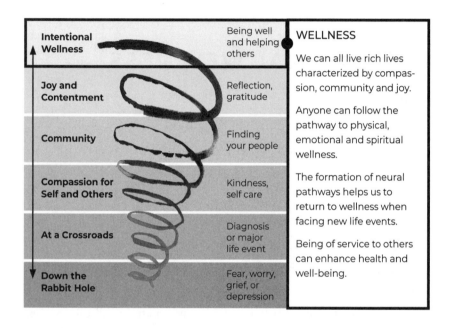

Mallika Chopra, daughter of the well-known Deepak Chopra, discusses a life with intention both in her book and in her 2020 TEDx talk. In her book *Living With Intent: My Somewhat Messy Journey to Purpose, Peace, and Joy*, she describes intentions as "expressions of who we aspire to be as individuals—physically, emotionally, spiritually…" To tap into our intentions, she suggests we must learn about our fears, insecurities, strengths, and passions.

Intentional wellness is more than being healthy. It is believing we are able to find wellness and ability when we face challenges, when illness occurs, and even at the end of our lives.

CREATING A PLAN

Planning helps us to define our priorities and get clear on our intentions. Some people can easily envision their best life and path in their heads; others prefer to create a written plan that they can hold in their hands. Both ways work. The important part is to understand how you want your life to go. If this process feels daunting to you, many tools are available to help plan. In previous chapters, you may have started writing in a notebook or a gratitude journal, and this might form the basis for your planning. ECalendars, online reminders, vision boards, journals and intentional life plans can all assist you, and lend guidance and structure.

Wouldn't it be lovely if someone could hand out maps with instructions to life's biggest challenges? A nice graphic depicting the right way to go about a challenging new journey? It might take some of the fun out of the ride but it sure would add confidence to finding a way through.

There are several intentional life plans that you can find online by searching, or you can create your own version, in as creative a form as you want. It's for you, so let it reflect your thoughts. Here are some of the questions you'll want to ask yourself and make a record on paper or online if you create an intentional life plan.

Who are the most important people to you? Imagine the people you feel closest to, for example, your children or grandchildren. Have you found tangible, lasting ways to show your connection to them? How will you honor those relationships? How might that change as you age? As your chronic illness progresses?

Where do you want to live, both now and in the future? Have you always wanted to live for a year, for example, on a houseboat? Do you want to be near the ocean or the mountains? What accommodations will you need? How might you make this dream happen? If your dream seems out of reach, are there other measures you can take such as short day trips to your favorite locations or trading house-sitting with friends?

How do you want to spend your days? What will you do for fun? Are there hobbies you wish to pursue?

Do you have a budget? What is your plan, money-wise? Do you have (or want) a financial advisor? Your financial future is outside the scope of this book. Whole sections of libraries are devoted to this topic. We don't claim to have the answers here.

What goals do you have? How will you work to make them happen? Some examples of goals include finally writing that novel, creating a blog, learning new recipes, traveling to a state park that you have always wanted to visit, tracing your DNA genealogy, or volunteering for any number of causes. The list is endless.

If you have a hard time answering some of these questions, that's okay. You can make it your task to start finding some answers. What do you want to do with your life? You are the only one who knows.

Pause to reflect: *Do you have ideas you want to try and a plan to do so? What is preventing you from exploring these ideas? Are there some "out of the box" ways to achieve your goals or finance them?*

Planner: Kat

For much of my life I planned everything. It was my way of navigating and making sense of my world. As a child, I loved writing things on the calendar, family birthdays, holidays, field trips and school events. As a high school student, I was never without my planner. It helped me to keep in order school and work schedules, swim meets, volleyball practice, choir rehearsals and the like. I was lost without my planner and spent many hours weekly "maintaining" my schedule.

I invested a great deal of time setting goals and making lists to achieve my goals. I was always looking to the next horizon. I studied hard and held multiple part time jobs while a full-time college student.

In my professional life, I lived by my planner. I even called it "my brain." When many of my colleagues switched to digital calendars on their phones or desktop computers, I could still be found most mornings reviewing "my brain" over my morning cup of tea. It was the first thing out onto my desk at the office or call room and the last thing put into my bag going home.

I think my attention to and interest in my planner was a symbolic reflection of me. My need to make order out of chaos and to feel in control of my life. This process leant comfort and reassurance that I could plan the events in my world, that perhaps I could control the uncontrollable. Perhaps the process lulled me into a false sense of order. The lists and the events were perpetual and reinforced the process of plan: do, go, list, produce, achieve, and repeat. The planner was a great tool for the "to do" but not one to learn "to be."

With my diagnosis came the opportunity to reevaluate the hamster wheel I was running on. Was it healthy? Could my demanding, sometimes ridiculous, hours co-exist with listening to my body and self-care? For me, the answer was a resounding no. It was time for a new plan.

WHEN THE PLAN CHANGES

We all possess built-in wisdom and knowledge about navigating challenges even when we must create and recreate our plans. We do not have a prescription for instant resilience but have developed this wellness model to be helpful in our journey to living resilient lives. It can lead to a feeling of chronic, sustained well-being, and when practiced, it can help you find your way back when facing new challenges.

At some point, many of our best-laid plans are disrupted. When this happens, it is a time that can lead to analysis. It is a time when many of us realize that we have little control over our world. It is a period of taking stock of life's essentials at a tipping point.

As previously discussed, grief is an important and necessary process when learning of a new diagnosis. Grieving is a necessary part of growing and ultimately learning to stay in the present moment to find joy and contentment.

HANDLING THE UNEXPECTED

Learning about changing your brain and practicing mindfulness is a big step towards resilience. Seeking and finding joy in life has also proven hugely important to well-being. Yet all skills can face challenges.

Challenges like a global pandemic. The world's response to the COVID-19 virus shut down life as we knew it. Quarantine, social distancing, an overnight shift from an active, outwardly facing lifestyle to one of strictly limited interaction with the world outside of one's own home.

This was a time of huge challenge on multiple levels. Fear of the unknown can become a pervasive emotion in this circumstance. For those who have been working at re-training their brains to stay in the present moment may be a step ahead of the curve in finding a way to stay sane in unexpected times.

Many of us with a chronic illness were classified as a high-risk group during the outbreak. Though Parkinson's is not a disease of the immune system, it can affect one's ability to effectively use muscles to properly clear airways, even in the early stages of the disease. In the case of COVID-19 that affects the respiratory tract, this meant we were more at risk of contracting the virus.

Never was it more a test of staying in the moment when other thoughts threatened to take over. "Are my children at risk? My daughter is a healthcare worker and ill and I cannot be with her. How do I keep safe? What if…?" The pervasive fears that we could all experience during unprecedented times of a global pandemic teased the outer reaches of our minds.

Remembering how to escape the rabbit hole thinking and keeping thoughts present in the moment were strategies that served us well during the unknown times of the pandemic.

Hands: Kat

I was getting used to the idea that I had Parkinson's disease, maybe even hitting a bit of a stride—writing a blog, speaking, accepting my transition to medical leave when a new challenge came with a new diagnosis—dystonia, which is abnormal contraction of muscles that is likely caused by a lack of dopamine in the brain. Not everyone with Parkinson's will experience dystonia. It is more common among those diagnosed with young onset. Many people will experience it in their feet, hands are less often affected. Both of my hands are affected.

After leaving my midwifery career, I struggled to redefine myself and learned new skills, but most of them rely on the use of my hands—painting, writing, boxing.

Dystonia took me by surprise. It was painful and made it more challenging to do all the things I had just learned to do. It felt "unfair," hadn't I given up enough? How do I keep going? Why me? It was a blow for sure. The grief set in again and thoughts led down the rabbit hole.

I grieved for the way I had learned to use my hands. I was angry that I was in pain and not able to do the things I love. I hurt. I often needed strong muscle relaxants to help ease the cramping pain so I could sleep. It was a low time.

Then after a few weeks, I noticed that I was learning new ways to paint. I learned new dictation software on my phone, computer and in my car to help with writing. I was adapting, learning to focus again on what I could do, and finding new ways to do what I love. I felt hope and found joy again. It almost surprised me going through the process that I was able to get back to joy so quickly after the initial blow.

The framework that developed after Sawyer's diagnosis helped me find wellness and joy after my own diagnosis. I learned to practice mindfulness and meditation and exercised often. My boxing community and support group helped me as I faced the new challenge of pain from dystonia. Perhaps most helpful was keeping my thoughts focused on what I could still do. I could speak, I could write and paint in different ways, and the garbage truck still came every Wednesday morning. My focus and previous practice had laid down pathways in my brain that allowed me to refocus my thoughts and to be well.

The dystonia is a part of my experience, an uninvited unexpected painful complication, but I was slowly finding joy again. I was able to use my practice of gratitude and found the way back to acceptance and compassion. It was a powerful example of how training my brain to lean into my abilities and joy helped me to find my way back after grieving. Like a muscle remembering how to ride a bike, it came back quickly.

When my aunt heard about my dystonia, she sent me a card describing the Japanese tradition and art of filling cracks in china with gold. Making that which is broken a unique treasure. This was a particularly special card to receive from my aunt who has had Rheumatoid arthritis for over 20 years. She added the note "perhaps we are all golden."

Getting On With Life: Nancy

When I met my neurologist, she told me that, one day, my Parkinson's would be just one component of who I am. I couldn't believe that would ever be true, but there are days, lots of days, when it is.

My husband and I decided to quit postponing the things we wanted to do. We wanted to see the lakes outside of Helsinki, the old town of Tallinn in Estonia, and the Arctic terns in Iceland. I worked with my coach to come up with an exercise plan that I could do in a hotel room. I packed a folding pair of walking sticks and made sure I always traveled with a good pair of walking shoes. Through a series of misadventures where I towed my suitcase through rain and mud and train stations, I learned to take the lightest amount of luggage so that I could carry it myself if necessary. You never know what unexpected events will happen.

Because I was newly diagnosed, I had a lot of fear when I started traveling again. If we went walking, I was afraid of losing my balance or falling. The truth was that I was just as afraid of looking awkward, of being too stiff, or not being able to walk. Could I still travel? The answer was a resounding yes. There were hurdles to take one at a time, but none proved insurmountable. I learned to not let fear of the unknown cause me to quit doing the things I love.

PROGRESSIVE DISEASE

As life progresses, we gather experiences and plan for what is ahead. With Parkinson's disease, that also means we experience disease progression. No matter the pace, a progressive disease eventually worsens. We exercise hard and often. We surround ourselves with supportive friends. We stay current on the research; we take our medications. We check all the boxes, we jump through all the hoops, and yet our symptoms take more energy to manage. The days slowly fill with more attention to the disease. We may need more medicine or new ones, and even brain surgery can be recommended to treat symptoms.

In our culture, we are used to being told how to fix what is wrong with us. If you have a headache, take an aspirin. If you break a limb, you get a cast, follow a plan, and get better. Cancer? Treat it, fight, get to the cure. The reality is that there is not a way to beat a disease that is incurable. Treatments are often aimed at a moving, changing target that varies from person to person. Acceptance and re-framing are key to riding the waves of chronic illness.

With each change or progression noticed, a bit of grief occurs. We feel the loss, and this grief and sadness are important to honor. The tricky part is to not allow yourself to stay too long in sadness. Look for your way back to wellness. Your tools —compassion, gratitude and mindfulness, community, joy, and intention— can be your anchor.

Each step of the way, we surrender a bit more of our old normal, grieve for it, succumb, and eventually accept the new normal. The other option is to stay in a state of perpetual grief and dread, the rabbit hole. If you can open yourself up to grieve over all that you have lost, and still see the glimmer of self-compassion on your horizon, you can climb out of the rabbit hole and back to wellness.

Our wellness spiral offers an alternative to staying lost. It is a cycle of symptoms, changing, grief/loss, re-evaluation, acceptance, and joy.

Maybe you have heard this saying that is attributed to an anonymous beach surfer: "Sometimes you just have to ride the wave you're given." The waves we ride are from the highs of a great day to the lows of accepting progression in disease. The waves continue to come. We ride as long as we can.

There are times when the changes crashing around us feel very close to home, for example, during the holidays. It's that time of year when we remember family rituals like going for walks in the snow and visiting with out-of-town guests. We cannot help but notice that another year has passed in the progression of our disease. This happened to Kat when she was busily preparing Thanksgiving dinner and realized that her hands and fingers were not going to allow her to peel potatoes. It may seem like a small thing that someone else can easily step in and do, but it is the task that she has always done. She asked her son and daughters to help, and they graciously took over without any fuss. It was the passing of the torch for this small task, and it symbolized a beginning of change.

We have learned to be grateful that we are alive to be able to share the holidays with family. We are grateful to receive help from our adult children to do tasks like making mashed potatoes. There is a slow transfer to the next generation. It is the beginning of grace as we learn to let go.

END OF LIFE WELLNESS

Life is finite. It is up to each of us to navigate the progression of age and disease. There is room for both progression and wellness. Your mind and your ability to use a practice of mindfulness and gratitude to get out of the rabbit hole can shape how you will navigate the end of your life. It may seem odd that a book about wellness and joy also includes a discussion about end of life and death. We pose, however, that a life practice of wellness can prepare one for death with intention and empowerment.

In his book, *Being Mortal: Medicine and What Matters in the End*, the author Atul Gawande, a palliative care physician, discusses the decisions that can lead to expensive, life-prolonging treatments that may not prolong quality of life. He believes that medicine has lost sight of easing suffering in its goal to treat disease at all costs. Sometimes the best interest of the patient and family can be doing nothing but easing pain. Hospice and palliative providers are experts at holistic care. If we want input on how the end of our lives are managed, we must have discussions early to determine what desires are at the end of life. There are legal tools to help document what you want and don't want to happen if life-threatening events occur.

Physician Orders for Life Sustaining Treatment (POLST) is a documented plan which must be filled out by you and signed by your physician. It is usually kept in a prominent place in a home, like the refrigerator door, to be shared with first responders as needed. It lists your desired wishes for initiation of life-saving measures when you are near the end of life. A Power of Attorney (POA) document expresses who can make decisions on your behalf if you are no longer able to communicate your wishes to your care team. There is a POA for medical and a POA for finances. Having these documents completed and accessible on demand can greatly relieve stress and anxiety in the twilight days.

In the last decade, the conversations around death and dying have been explored in new ways. For example, death cafes are a compassionate place where people, often strangers, gather to eat, drink, and discuss death. The get-togethers allow, literally or virtually, for honest discussions. What life saving measures do we want taken? How to fill out a POLST? How to have honest communication with your loved ones about your desires? How can we build community and support end of life discussions and decisions? You can find more information, including locations for the nearest death cafes, at https://deathcafe.com/.

Your provider, hospital or clinic will have information available about advanced directives. Be sure to inquire about these and make your desires known and document them. That way everyone involved knows ahead of time how to honor your final wishes.

Meet Our Friends: Harry and Kerry Rae

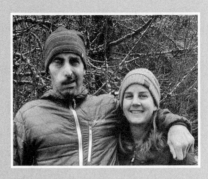

Six months after his Parkinson's diagnosis at age 47, Harry and his wife Kerry Rae sold everything they owned to travel around South America for ten months. Several years later, his symptoms were progressing and impacting his ability to work and enjoy life enough so that Harry's neurologist suggested having surgery—deep brain stimulation—to hopefully help with his movement difficulties and side effects from medication. He was reluctant but felt he had exhausted his medication options and was struggling with rigidity, dystonia, and severe dyskinesia.

Harry underwent deep brain stimulation (DBS) surgery in December of 2017. During surgery there was a complication, and he suffered a massive stroke. It was a devastating blow.

The stroke left him completely insensate on his left side, from head to toe, and he lost the ability to see and hear on his right side. Disabled and confined to a wheelchair, he was also severely affected by Parkinson's.

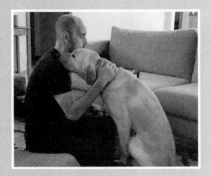

Harry worked tirelessly at his physical and occupational therapy with hopes to regain his independence. Ras, Harry's trained service dog, played a crucial role in his day-to-day life, and he was a crowd favorite at Parkinson's fundraising walks.

Harry passed away in 2021. His phenomenal inner strength, grit, and quest for adventure made him a beacon of light and resilience. Harry and Kerry Rae represent the ability to love unconditionally and overcome obstacles that seem insurmountable in life and in death. Kerry Rae continues to carry their combined strength and his memory. ✳

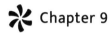 Chapter 9

HEALTH CARE TEAM

"If you want to go fast, go alone. If you want to go far, go together."

—AFRICAN PROVERB

YOUR HEALTH CARE TEAM will likely include your care partner and a cadre of health professionals and practitioners. Each plays a different role in your care community. Some team members are neurologists or movement disorder specialists or technicians who help diagnose disease. Others treat symptoms or care for your physical and emotional needs. We look at this as a team effort since all of these individual actions interact and affect your state of health.

There are usually many options when choosing members of your care team. As you build your team, find out who is affordable and recommended by those you trust. Read reviews and ask around for input from others. You can interview potential providers for what they do. It is important to remember that you are hiring them to help care for you. Besides learning about their skills, be sure to find out what charges to expect and if they are covered by your insurance plan.

In addition to your primary care doctor and medical specialists, your care team might include:

- Mental health therapists
- A member of the clergy
- Pharmacist
- Occupational therapist
- Physical therapist
- Massage therapist
- Dietitian

- Chiropractor
- Acupuncturist
- Naturopath
- Women's health professional
- Family and friends
- Care partner

It is important to create an atmosphere of open communication with the primary members of your care team. If someone does not seem to be listening to or understanding you, keep trying. Be sure to speak up for yourself. Communication, to be effective, must flow both ways. You must make it a priority to share with others how you are feeling, which tools are helping, which don't seem to be, and to listen to their response. If a new symptom comes to light, it is important to let others know, even though it can sometimes be a challenge to be so forthcoming.

You can be the one who sets the stage for effective communication. It's important because the medical professionals who share in your care may work at different facilities and for different agencies, but they may share responsibilities for common face-to-face tasks such as acting as your health coach, reconciling your medications, and reviewing test results and other findings with you and your family, as well as non-face-to-face tasks such as telephone and email communication, processing clinical reminders, and handling the ever-present paperwork (Kim, L., et al, 2019). There is a heightened risk of something falling through the cracks—something important and possibly life altering—if you haven't created a climate of direct and open communication.

YOUR PRIMARY CARE PROVIDER (PCP)

Your PCP will be a key player in the care you receive. They may be a nurse practitioner, a physician's assistant, a family practice physician, or an internist. They should be kept informed about the specialists you are seeing. Some insurances will require that you see them first to get a referral for specialized care. It is an industry standard that specialists send a report to your primary care after seeing you and making recommendations. If you can self-refer to specialty care, it will be important that you keep your primary care up to date about who you are scheduling with and be sure the specialist sends a report to your PCP.

Your PCP will also be the one you need to see for other health related challenges such as upper respiratory infections, sprained or strained muscles, and preventative care such as routine annual exams. Management of ongoing chronic health challenges that are under control are also managed by a PCP.

For those of you in rural areas that do not have nearby options for specialty care, it may require a drive and consultation with a specialist initially to recommend a plan of care. This plan will then be executed by you and your PCP, or you can inquire about the option to use telehealth. It is now an option with some health care systems to offer appointments over an internet call or live chat. This opens greater opportunities for everyone to access the care that best suits their needs, regardless of their geography.

OTHER HEALTH CARE PROVIDERS

Feeling comfortable with your health care team is important. For a long time, we have lived in a culture that reveres physicians and health care providers. When we are ill, we go to them to "heal" us. We accept any recommendation without question because we trust their knowledge and we want to feel well. With the creation of modern antibiotics, we have good reason to revere our "healers." Bacterial infections that once were life threatening are suddenly cured with tablets. This feels miraculous and contributes to the "doctor knows best" mentality.

The hero worship of care providers, however, has led many to forget that these are professionals we hire to share their advice and knowledge about disease and wellness. Ultimately, it is up to us, the person managing life with a diagnosis, to decide how, when and if to integrate advice and prescription.

A recent paper discusses the importance of a model that puts the patient in the center of the team. From the patient there are others (a community) that radiates from them. Care partners, children, physicians, other specialty care providers all surround the patient. As you move into a life of intentional wellness it will likely change the way you interact with your care team. Remembering that you are central to every decision and choice can be an important shift in thinking in today's healthcare climate (Bloem et al, 2020).

Seeking out providers and care team members is an important task for us all. Being intentional when selecting your team will enhance your journey navigating a chronic illness. Developing rapport and mutual respect are key to feeling comfortable and supported.

Fear can affect our perception of pain and tension. If we are able to arm ourselves with knowledge, we can enhance our quality of life, decrease our tension, and pain, and feel greater confidence in ourselves and our decisions.

Helpful tips to consider adding to your pre-appointment routine include:

- Make a list of items you want to discuss and encourage your care partner to do the same. Review with each other both lists before you go to the appointment.

- Take another person with you to your appointment.

- If it is not possible to have someone accompany you, ask if recording advice on a phone is ok with your care provider, or ask them to detail instructions on the printed visit summary to take home with you.

- Consider telehealth visits to have another person with you during visits.

Having another person hear, help remember, and even take notes about what is discussed in your appointment can help you to focus. It can be comforting to know you have another to check in about the specifics, especially when discussing changes to your routine. During the coronavirus quarantine, this became a real challenge, so we have encouraged people to record the visit on a cell phone to be able to reflect about what was discussed. If you want to use a recording, you must be sure to let the provider know and have their permission to record the conversation before doing so. Having access to your electronic medical record, or EMR, can also help track recommendations and changes discussed at visits.

Doing some preparation before you go to your visit can set you up for getting the most out of your time with your providers. As already discussed, you and your care partner can prepare for appointments by setting aside some time to discuss and check in about how treatments and symptoms are going. It is also important to understand what certain providers will manage and treat. This aspect of health care is one the most confusing pieces when you first have a team helping to take care of you.

Your neurologist, hopefully one that specializes in movement disorders, will be the one assessing and treating your nervous system. They will manage the medications you take to replace the dopamine that your body no longer makes. They will ask you to show them how your body is moving and discuss with you your impression of how you are doing. Their exam and expertise are focused on Parkinson's symptoms and treatment.

For those of us with Parkinson's disease, we know there are many symptoms, motor (movement) and non-motor. Your neurologist may not be the one who will help manage many of the non-motor symptoms. An example can be if you are having trouble with choking or not swallowing your food well. For this symptom, you will likely be referred to a doctor that specializes in disorders of the ear, nose, and throat. These are the experts in assessing what is happening with your swallowing and can make recommendations for treatment in the most informed way. As a patient, it can be frustrating to know that Parkinson's is causing a problem, but you may need many different specialists to manage the symptoms.

It is important to remember which provider manages what part of your health care. It may not be realistic for you to expect your neurologist to manage other chronic health conditions. Ask questions about who does what. Remember that you remain in charge of your team.

MAKING INFORMED DECISIONS

You are the leader, the captain, the Chief Executive Officer, the president of your care team. If a member of your team is not working well for you, find someone new. Talk with others whose approach to health is similar to yours. Read about them and their philosophy in literature about the practice, or a bio online. Interview providers. Many have free get-acquainted or meet the provider visits. Take a list of questions. It is okay to move to another provider if you do not feel comfortable having a dialogue with someone.

There are benefits, alternatives, and risks (remember BAR?) to every decision that is made. It is important to consider all three aspects before you conclude what is best for you when making decisions about your health care and treatment. Be curious about a new option. Discuss the BAR with your provider, ask questions. Seek opinions of others trying new things. For many people, knowledge about their experience helps empower decision-making and makes adherence to a new regiment easier.

Consider the qualities you admire in the people you care about. Are they inquisitive, intellectual, talkative, good listeners, outspoken, quiet? It is OK and expected to seek out providers that share some of these qualities.

It is easy to feel overwhelmed by pills and procedures when you are managing a chronic health issue. When asked "Is this really necessary" by their patients, thirty percent of physicians replied that "no, it (the proposed intervention) was not medically necessary." However, many physicians feel much pressure from consumers, or patients, to "do something" to help their condition. When patients ask the questions "Is this necessary? What are the benefits, alternatives and risks?" 20% will change their original plan of action (Mjåset, 2019). When we collect information and learn to make informed decisions, it can impact how we feel about making our decision, our health, and our futures.

Pause to reflect: *Are you satisfied with your relationships with your team? If not, what changes can you make?*

MEDICATION

Perhaps one of the biggest decisions you will consider is starting medication. Medication is one way to treat symptoms. In order to optimize your health and well-being, you and your prescribing provider must work together when considering starting a medication, changing a dose, or stopping a medication. It can be dangerous to suddenly stop or change a dosage of some medicines. Be sure to consult before you do so.

If, or when to start medication is a personal choice. We urge you to have a full understanding of each recommended medicine and of the implications of making your choice. There are benefits, alternatives, and risks in starting anything new. It is important to seek the information you need to make an informed decision. Ask your prescribing provider questions. Ask about potential side effects. Ask about what to expect with the timing of relief with a new dose or new medicine. Read labels and ask trusted sources of information. Once you start, it will be important to keep close track of the medications you are taking and the dosage.

Make sure that any medication you take can be absorbed by your body as fully as possible. Proper hydration helps all of our bodies to function optimally. It is also important to help your medication work the way it is intended. Try to slowly drink a full glass of water every time you swallow pills—no quick gulps because you are in a hurry. Check your nutrition and the food you eat to make sure that you are not consuming protein at a time that interferes with the absorption of some medicines in your stomach. You can work with your doctor to find the best times and habits for you.

The gold standard medication to treat symptoms of Parkinson's is carbidopa-levodopa (Sinemet is a common brand name). It is a tried-and-true medicine effective in treating tremors and muscle rigidity. Taking large amounts of levodopa over prolonged periods of time can lead to long-term side effects that involve involuntary muscle movements called dyskinesia. It can also become less and less effective for shorter periods of time. However, it is the best medication we have at the moment. There are some medications that can help minimize side effects and others that can help with the periods of time that carbidopa-levodopa is less effective.

A class of medications called dopamine agonists is used sometimes as front-line treatment in younger patients with Parkinson's disease, or as an adjunct to help with off periods. Off periods can occur when your carbidopa/levodopa dose wears off before the next dose is taken, or when medication doesn't kick in when it should. The dopamine agonists enhance existing dopamine and can impact your pleasure control center in the brain. Many people use these medications with success to remediate their symptoms, many use it with small side effects and others have reported significant side effects, including hyper-sexuality, insomnia, and compulsive behaviors such as spending, gambling, and overeating.

Dopamine agonists are associated with Impulse Control Disorders (ICDs). The higher the dose of the dopamine agonist and/or the longer the frequency, the higher the risk of developing ICDs. It is important to discuss how you and your care partner will check in about the potential side effects and when to call your provider. It can often be the care partner that notices changing behaviors.

We want to emphasize that you are in charge of your health and that includes what medications you chose and when to take them. There is some evidence that suggests taking medication earlier in the disease process may lengthen the window of time you experience better treatment of symptoms. The theory is that the more the disease progresses, the higher the dose of medicine it takes to help mitigate the symptoms. The more medication, the higher the risk of side effects. Balancing the risks of complications with timing of when the medicine will be most effective often takes trial, error, patience, a healthy sense of humor, and lots of self-compassion.

A surgical treatment for Parkinson's symptoms called deep brain stimulation, or DBS, involves putting electrodes into the brain. A rechargeable battery unit is also surgically implanted in the chest cavity near the collarbone. Electrodes can be placed on one or both sides of the brain, and small electrical impulses stimulate areas of the brain that help to decrease many of the motor symptoms impacted by Parkinson's. DBS is sometimes called the pacemaker for the brain. It is a brain surgery and comes with the usual risks for any surgical procedure in the brain. This surgery is usually recommended when symptoms are no longer well-controlled with medications or if the side effects are impacting quality of life.

There is not a prescribed right way to go about treatment. The medications available help with many symptoms but do not cure the disease, and not everyone with Parkinson's will experience relief of symptoms with these medications or treatments.

What can impact a sense of wellness is how much one feels in control of the process of how, when, or whether to take medicine, to have surgery, or to try other options. Having a provider who is willing to be your partner on the journey of disease management and one whom you trust is crucial to how you will feel moving forward with new interventions. In other words, you are likely to feel better about yourself if you play an active role in treatment rather than feeling that you are a passive participant in your journey.

When you take medications regularly, it is important to talk to your prescribers about potential drug interactions. Insist that your doctor provide a regular evaluation on the dosage and the need for all medicines that you take.

If you have unusual symptoms, document them and don't hesitate to reach out to a medical professional. Don't assume that all changes or new symptoms are related to your Parkinson's disease medications or to progression of the disease. We have heard about people having drug interactions or developing another health issue that they assumed, wrongly, was caused by their Parkinson's disease.

A trusted team member to consult can be your pharmacist. You can work toward establishing a relationship with a pharmacy by getting your prescriptions filled at the same place consistently, and by asking questions, when you have them, of the pharmacists. For example, your pharmacist will be able to advise if you require an over-the-counter analgesic or cold medication that is compatible with your prescription medications. It is important to consult before using other medications, even over the counter medications and supplements.

ONE TREATMENT AT A TIME

Trying multiple treatment methods at the same time can be confusing and harmful. If you are introducing more than one treatment and you experience a benefit or a complication, it is impossible to know which treatment or intervention is helping or hindering the process. Though you may be tempted to do it all, be cautioned that it is not in your best interest to try it all at once.

It may be helpful to look at the process of treatments in a methodical way. Jot down the dates you start a process or new treatment and keep notes about what you experience. You can even make a place for it in your calendar. This applies to supplements, over-the counter medications, and prescriptions. As you collect the information and notice trends, it can further inform you and your care team about which approach is helping you the most.

There are some great resources available to track medications and to prepare you for meeting with your provider both digital and paper versions. The *Every Victory Counts* manual from the Davis Phinney Foundation outlines ways to prepare for appointments with your neurologist or provider.

Preparing for your appointment will help you to get the most out of the short time you have with your provider. Letting them know right away that you have some questions is important; don't wait until the end of the appointment. That way they know to make time for your questions. It also signals to the provider that you are invested in your care and respect their time.

It is important to keep your care team informed about changes in your treatment plan or in what you are trying in terms of medication. Many today are using supplemental sources to round out or add to their health regimen. Supplements are included in those things you need to discuss with your provider. Bringing notes to appointments can make your visits more efficient. Printing out a copy of your findings can help your provider understand your experience and guide treatment decisions.

THE PATIENT PERSPECTIVE

Keeping informed in today's world with the overabundance of information outlets can seem a daunting task. Yet, for many of us, being informed about our health is central to being able to make intentional decisions about how we stay healthy and manage illness and aging.

We recommend that you carry a small notebook or paper or make a notation in your smartphone to keep notes about any topics that catch your interest. Write it down as soon as you can while the information is still fresh. Describe who told you or where you first heard about it. You can make a note online or send yourself a text.

Keep an informed eye on what's being reported in the media. Most online and broadcast stations keep an index of previous subjects. If there is a newly published book being publicized, you can check websites that review books on shows like *Good Morning America*, *the Today Show*, *NPR*, Public Radio programs, and many more. If a magazine article looks useful, use your cellphone to take a photo of the article and snap the cover of the magazine that shows the date or edition. If it isn't a magazine that you normally have access to, you can check with your library to see if they can get a copy of the article for you.

Sometimes we overhear snippets of people talking, say, at the gym. Try to capture what you do know, or what it sounded like, to the best of your ability. Even if you don't know all the details, save what you do know. The important thing is to get enough information so that you can follow up if it is a topic of interest.

Once you have the article or report in your hands, be sure to evaluate any research results carefully. You will need to thoughtfully read the research that interests you. Studies can be flawed, or worse, make claims that their own research does not support. Be cautious about believing any articles that make outrageous claims. You will want to read and think carefully about what's being presented. Here are some questions you can ask.

Given your current level of knowledge, does the new information seem reasonable and believable to you?

- Is the source of the information legitimate?
- Who funded the study or trial? Do you trust them?
- How many people were studied? Does it seem like a large enough sample size?
- If it's a new medicine, what trial stage is it in? Has it gone through rigorous testing and human trials?

Keep track of all the questions you have. It's easy to fall for a false promise when one is eager for a cure. Sift through to find what is true for you based on the symptoms you are experiencing. Consider focusing on information published by trusted organizations such as the Parkinson's Foundation, Michael J Fox Foundation, Davis Phinney Foundation, and World Parkinson Coalition.

Find out who the publisher is whenever you are reading about new studies. For example, research published about drug trials that are funded by drug companies may have biased results, whereas peer-reviewed clinical journals such as the Journal of the American Medical Society or the British Medical Journal are typically well-known, reliable sources.

THE PROVIDER PERSPECTIVE

Your healthcare team will also be keeping up to date. A part of ongoing licensure for providers includes continuing medical education (CME). CME can be achieved by reading articles in medical journals, attending conferences where new research is being presented, and/or completing coursework. In other words, it is reasonable to expect your providers to stay current with new developments in the field.

It is important to understand, however, that it is not considered good practice to change disease management based on a single outcome of a single trial. For patients, that can prove frustrating at times. We hear about some great new breakthrough that seemed to relieve symptoms and our provider is not ready to try it. From the provider perspective it can be dangerous and costly to change practice based on single study outcomes. Best practice dictates that a study be duplicated multiple times to ensure safety and efficacy before becoming a new best practice and being widely recommended by healthcare providers.

Caution and patience are important traits when helping to care for patients. Again, the partnership between patient and provider will prove to be a critical part of navigating intentional wellness. Open communication is the foundation of navigating this important relationship between you and your team.

Meet Our Friend: Claudia

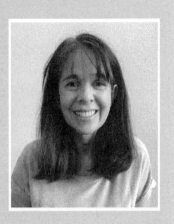

Claudia inspires and motivates us. She stays up with the latest research about exercise and works with her care team to keep in the best health. She keeps us honest with our timing and is ever watchful to keep our heart rates up in the high intensity level for at least 30 minutes. We know that studies recommend this level of intensity, and she holds us to it.

Claudia was diagnosed with Parkinson's at the age of 50 and works harder than anyone else at our ladies' bootcamp on Saturday mornings. She cheers us to work hard, run fast, punch hard and keep going. Her enthusiasm and fierce attack on the punching bags prompts us to work that much harder.

She is all heart and little filter. Her summary of a complex research presentation about alpha-synuclein cells using an analogy to clumping pasta in the brain left us in hysterics. She said, "To summarize, spaghetti, linguini, we are all f@#*^ed!"

Originally from Mexico, Claudia moved to the states with her family over a decade ago. She is driven to stay in Oregon due to the medical and social resources here in the United States. We hope Claudia will stay with us because we can't imagine our workouts without her. ✳

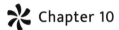 Chapter 10

BEING WELL

"For there is always light, if only we're brave enough to see it."
—National Youth Poet Laureate Amanda
Gorman during the 2020 inauguration
ceremony.

WE HOPE THAT OUR wellness spiral has helped you think about the journey to wellness, and that you continue to find new ways to live a joyful and contented life. None of us have been promised a straight or easy path forward to wellness, but even if you get sidetracked, there are many places along the spiral for you to step back in and continue your journey.

Have you integrated some new elements such as mindfulness, gratitude, and community into your way of being? Each of us has our own wisdom and ability to make choices that best fit into our individual lives. Your commitment to your intentional wellness practice, your role in helping others, and your capacity to experience hope and joy will help you navigate more of your journey.

If you find yourself in a rabbit hole—you are discouraged or anxious or unable to work on your best behalf—it is an opportunity to act with compassion. Treat yourself as you would a loved one who is suffering. Believe that you deserve to have joy, exactly like other people on this planet do. Use writing or art to express how you are feeling. If it helps you get started in a journal, you can use a compassionate prompt such as, "What do I need at this moment?"

If you are at a major life event or crossroads, remember that you can try a mindfulness-based program such as guided meditation, breathing exercises or other forms of relaxation. You can do this alone or with a group. Studies show that an increase in mindfulness practice can improve your relationships and self-confidence in managing disease. If you join a group mindfulness-based program, you have the potential for increasing both your sense of control over your reactions to disease symptoms as well as your social connectedness (Vandenberg, 2019).

Finally, if you are lonely, reach out to someone in your community. Opening yourself up to meet and get to know other people can chase away loneliness, both yours and theirs. It may be your community that allows you to start new behaviors in your practice of intentional wellness. In her book, Mallika Chopra shares the value of having a village. She writes, "when people support one another, it creates momentum, instills confidence and inspires action to take necessary steps to change."

On good days, nothing seems too hard. We joyously go about our routine with full force. On other days, we tell ourselves that all we must do is show up to an engagement or event that we have committed to doing. Once there, we can muster the energy to participate and maybe engage fully.

Sometimes showing up is the best you can do. When energy wains, it takes all the days' effort just to exist. Because fatigue is so unpredictable, it is one of the biggest challenges with Parkinson's disease.

It can be difficult to stay motivated to do all the things we know are important to our wellness, such as exercising or showing up to participate in our community. Once relationships are established, which is a health benefit unto itself, it adds a new level of commitment to the process.

One of the ways we stay motivated is to remind ourselves that it is important to keep our commitments. We show up for one another. Our friends and fellow Parkinson's disease fighters rely on us. As a group, we are truly more than the sum of our parts. Together we face many symptoms. Without our relationships, we might very well withdraw and isolate ourselves. Together, we help each other show up and carry on the fight.

HELPING OTHERS

Do you want to spend time working, volunteering, contributing, or becoming an activist in the causes that matter to you? Volunteering can be a powerful way to feel vital and engaged, and many studies have shown that being a volunteer contributes to better health, both physically and mentally. People who volunteer report that they are more satisfied with their lives and rate their overall health as better (Lawton, 2021).

Helping others also can stimulate the pleasure centers in your brain. MRI studies have found that when we are giving to others in acts of altruism the same parts of the brain that respond to the pleasures of eating or having sex are activated (Filkowski, 2016). Acts of altruism can help others and increase our health and happiness.

If you choose to volunteer your time, it doesn't have to involve a long-term commitment or take a huge amount of time to create better physical and mental health outcomes. You may need to brainstorm ideas if your symptoms limit your abilities, but people with disabilities or chronic health conditions can still benefit greatly from volunteering. In fact, research has shown that there is a connection between volunteering and positive health. Adults with disabilities or health conditions ranging from hearing and vision loss to diabetes or digestive disorders all showed improvement after volunteering. Furthermore, people who volunteer are more likely to participate in preventive health screenings (Kim, E., 2016).

Giving, even in simple ways, can be helpful. Here are some ideas for getting out and helping others that can be done with little fanfare.

- Send a note or card to someone who is grieving the loss of a friend or a relative, or feeling lonely.

- Invite a friendly neighbor for a walk around the block.

- Offer to volunteer online if you can use a computer.

- If your body and hands are able, pick up along a street or harvest ripe fruit with a gleaners' organization that donates the bounty to food banks.

Volunteering has many surprising benefits. It can help you focus on other people, and it takes your mind off your own situation. Donating your time connects you to others and can help battle loneliness. When you participate, it's easier to get tips on local concerts, find the best deals on fresh vegetables, or where to get free vaccines. Being a volunteer connects you to other organizations and people. It also provides you with emotional support.

From the beginning of humankind, it has been known that we reap benefits while doing for others. Many have been quoted saying that helping others can make you happier and provide purpose for living:

> *If you want happiness for an hour, take a nap. If you want happiness for a day, go fishing. If you want happiness for a year, inherit a fortune. If you want happiness for a lifetime, help somebody.* —Chinese proverb

> *For it is in giving that we receive.* —Saint Francis of Assisi

*The sole meaning of life is to serve
humanity.* —Leo Tolstoy

*We make a living by what we get; we make a life by what
we give.* —Winston Churchill

*Making money is a happiness; making other people happy
is a super happiness.* —Nobel Peace Prize recipient
Muhammad Yunus

*Giving back is as good for you as it is for those you
are helping, because giving gives you purpose. When
you have a purpose-driven life, you're a happier
person.* —Goldie Hawn

Being of Service: Kat

Finding myself and my inner calm with a gratitude practice and mindfulness led to inner peace for me. To continue to find balance, I also needed to find new ways to be of service in the world again.

Serving others is a part of my personality and always has been. There have been many opportunities, since my diagnosis, to use my provider and planning skills within the Parkinson's community. I have volunteered for several non-profit events and my work as a Davis Phinney Foundation Ambassador gives me an opportunity to be a resource for others with Parkinson's.

There have been times when I have taken a phone call not in the best "head space" about my own circumstances. By the time I'm off of the call I feel better. I helped somebody; I was able to share that having a diagnosis is not a death sentence. I word my philosophy and share it freely, "I seek joy in every day, and I refuse to be defined by any diagnosis." After saying the words out loud to another person, I remember my choice to walk in gratitude and joy. Having these interactions affords me the opportunity to lift myself up while trying to do the same for others.

When I am engaged with serving others, I am not focused on myself. This helps me to keep a much-needed perspective, be well, and remain intentional about where I focus my thoughts.

PARTICIPATING IN CLINICAL TRIALS

Research and clinical trials lie at the heart of all medical advances. Trials are supervised and must meet national standards. There are two main types, clinical trials, and observational studies. Clinical trials are performed to evaluate a new drug, surgery, or behavior, and observational studies look at individuals or measure certain outcomes.

You can find out about current clinical trials through Parkinson's support organizations, your neurologist's office, or online sites such as Fox Trial Finder at foxtrialfinder.org. The announcement for a trial will tell you what phase the trial is in, what the drug or behavior study will involve, and the criteria that the researchers have established for participation.

A clinical trial typically needs many people to enroll as test subjects. Before you decide to participate, be sure to get all the critical information you need to decide whether it is appropriate for you. There are risks you will want to understand before signing up to be a test subject, regardless of what the trial is studying.

Many clinical trials use a placebo to evaluate the effect of a new drug or therapy. A placebo can look and feel like it is real, but it delivers no active therapy. A good example of a placebo is a sugar pill that is substituted for a real pill. Even though people volunteering for a clinical trial understand that they might be receiving a placebo, it's not uncommon to experience a very real benefit from the placebo.

Thinking you'll feel better may change your brain chemistry or work in other ways to improve symptoms and quality of life. In fact, there's evidence that taking a placebo leads to changes in the brain, not unlike taking a dose of levodopa (Lidstone, 2014). Furthermore, people with Parkinson's experience a significant placebo effect. The reason why this happens isn't clear, but it may be because the release of dopamine plays a role in the brain's reward system. Because of this, Parkinson's clinical trials need to be designed so that they take the placebo effect into account.

Many people are proud to be part of a clinical trial as a way of giving back and helping to find a cure within the Parkinson's community. Some trials offer a stipend, or the chance to take a ground-breaking drug or its placebo. While you will always want to first consult with your doctors and care team, signing up to be in a trial is a personal decision and one that only you can make.

There are very few studies specifically discussing women and Parkinson's disease. The medicines prescribed for men and women were studied only in men. This is the case for most medicines for all diseases. Women and their ability to conceive a child makes scientists reluctant to use women in studies. It is important to realize that many people, not just women, are smaller and weigh less than the average 180-pound male in tests. Dosages for treatment must take into account all body types.

The hormonal differences in men and women are also not accounted for in most research. Women may need smaller doses and different medications to combat symptoms with menstrual cycles. There is emerging consensus that women who are menstruating require different dosages of Parkinson's medications the week leading up to and during their menses (Flanagan, 2021).

Getting involved in clinical trials can help us to have women better represented in the literature. Encouraging research on the female experience of Parkinson's will only strengthen our ability to understand our condition.

Pause to reflect: *Are there clinical trials in your area? Have you ever asked your provider about participation in a trial?*

ADVOCACY

The journey for us from midwife and librarian to women with Parkinson's, to speakers, all was a deep part of seeking, finding, and nurturing our wellness. Volunteering and helping others who were recently diagnosed helped us to find purpose in our own lives. It feels good and gives us joy.

We could never have guessed that we would be invited to be community leaders of a support group, learn to box, perform a dance number with a group of others with Parkinson's disease, or speak internationally about resilience. Though we are not grateful for the disease, we feel deeply thankful for the people we have met through our network of others with Parkinson's.

After the World Parkinson Congress in Portland in 2016, we set a goal to create and deliver a talk at the World Parkinson Congress in Japan in 2019. As we described earlier, the World Parkinson Congress is a unique and widely acclaimed conference that meets every three years. Its goal is to provide networking and knowledge sharing among the greatest stakeholders in Parkinson's disease. It is put on by the World Parkinson Coalition, headed by Eli Pollard.

We decided to expand our knowledge and research areas of interest to us. We spent time at the medical library reading about a broad range of things that lead us to the overriding topic of resilience. Our talk, "Resilience: Beyond a Diagnosis," was in the making. While we learned, we were also practicing a new way of being and of using our brains to find joy and wellness.

Over the course of 2018, we refined our talk and delivered it first to selected audiences in a series of six house parties. We then presented at large in Oregon, speaking at more than seven events throughout the state. We still are asked to share this talk at support groups in the state.

Going to Kyoto was a once-in-a-lifetime trip for both of us. It's hard to overstate how excited we were to have the opportunity to fly to Japan to speak at the World Parkinson Congress 2019.

Kyoto is a beautiful city. We rode the elevators to the top of the train station in amazement. The trains race by, clean and on time, and the signs are translated into English. Even as Westerners who did not speak the language, we had very little trouble getting around.

When we first started talking about going to the conference in Kyoto, we heard from several friends that they wanted to go along on the adventure. It was difficult for us to tell how serious people were until they all actually started making travel plans. All told, there were 13 people we knew traveling from Oregon to the congress. It was an amazing show of support and community.

Finding a Voice: Nancy

I came away from the congress having learned about current research on stem cells and the gut microbiome, and I felt I had found my voice in the conversation as a person living with chronic disease. I exchanged ideas with people from around the world. One night, we went to hear music performed by a group that included Michelle, our Portland friend profiled earlier, and her guitar-playing neurologist. For the finale, the audience flooded the stage with appreciation.

The World Parkinson Congress changed my relationship with Parkinson's disease. I am no longer just a person living with it, I also have an advocacy role. The Congress opened doors for me and renewed my hope in the future for people with Parkinson's disease.

The Start of a Movement: Kat

At the World Parkinson Congress in Kyoto, a small international group of attendees with young onset Parkinson's disease (YOPD) held a meeting to discuss advocacy. It was soon clear that many felt underrepresented in their respective countries and strongly desired a place to meet to discuss the unique needs of being young with Parkinson's disease. Many had little access to specialized neurology care or DBS. Many had little social support in their communities.

It was decided to organize a conference devoted to the needs of the YOPD people. No identification would be required to document age of diagnosis; it would be a self-selection process. It was at this meeting that I realized I needed to be a voice for this disease and contribute to this movement.

Unfortunately, COVID-19 made it impossible to meet. However, we are committed to moving forward and will meet at the next World Parkinson Congress with content specifically targeted for us.

In further advance of this cause, four movement disorder specialists, Ray Dorsey, Todd Sherer, Michael Okun and Bastiaan Bloem wrote an important book, *Ending Parkinson's Disease: A Prescription for Action*. It describes the need, in today's world of limited research dollars that are coveted by many groups, to organize and get loud to help push for better treatments and ultimately a cure for Parkinson's. The authors described the movements from the Susan B. Komen foundation and the AIDS activists of the 1980s as models for successful advocacy efforts.

As a direct result of the book, the PD Avengers patient advocacy group was formed by three YOPD advocates in Canada.

This group has a lofty goal of uniting one million voices rising to put an end to Parkinson's. The formation of the PD Avengers hopes to earn the right to more effectively lobby and receive research dollars to aid in better treatments and ultimately a cure. The group also wants to end the siloed work going on in research, especially in the United States. They aim to help bridge information and help organizations work together instead of competing, and to have patients involved in all levels of research and clinical trials, not only as test subjects.

It may take a revolution to cure a disease. Mindfulness makes more room for action. Hope fuels passion and community.

WHAT WE KNOW

- Having community prolongs life. We must stay engaged with others.

- Moving our bodies can ward off disease.

- Mindfulness and gratitude ground our intentions.

- Neural pathways focused on wellness and ability can help keep thoughts out of the rabbit hole.

- There is joy.

- You can be well with intention.

CURATING HOPE

Earlier on, we cautioned against becoming overly invested in a cure. We advised you not to waste too much time or energy waiting for the results of this or that promising research. Time is so precious. We stand by this advice. Don't put one day on hold. We wholeheartedly encourage you to desire a better outcome tomorrow, to want something wonderful to happen or be true. Being mindful and in the present will enhance life now and you can continue mindfulness when a cure arrives without sacrificing the present moment.

We invite you to hope, and to curate hope. By curating, we mean to take charge of it or organize; to pull together, sift through and select. To curate hope in one's life means looking within. Take the glimmers of hope that exist for you. Start to collect and care for the glimmers. Nurture them. Allow them to grow.

If your only hope is that of a cure, it leaves no room for hope now. We urge you to discover ways of collecting both joy and hope to maximize your life in the moment. This moment. Hope that grief will end. Hope that the practice of finding and collecting joy will be enough to draw you back to it when the small glimmers start to appear with a new symptom.

Hope can be what propels us out of the rabbit hole back to intentional wellness.

Pay attention to your glimmers of hope. Organize them, study them, remember them. Write them down, shout them out, dream about them, discuss them, write a poem about them, sing a song, you get the idea. It need not be a daunting task. Start small, let it build, and it will.

When you have an incurable progressive disease with no cure and few treatments, it can be hard to have hope. One can sink into excuses and give into self-defeating thoughts and actions. Keep hopeful thoughts handy when these thoughts start to creep in. Before long, those glimmers will glow and make it easier to keep the nagging dread out.

Hope can propel us forward to keep going. We hope for a good day, we hope that our children grow up safe and healthy, we hope for peace on earth. Hope is the promise of things yet to come.

WHERE THE JOURNEY CONTINUES

Being well means reflecting on the big picture and trusting the processes learned. Sharing our wellness spiral and our stories brings us joy and gratitude. We hope you are able to use some of the tools we have shared to live a life that is your best.

The project of co-writing this book enhanced our health and wellness. It gave us physiologic benefits of community, shared experience, and friendship. During the quarantine days, it also gave us focus and purpose. You can find ways to do the same.

You have everything you'll need to meet the life challenges that come your way. We've given you a system for looking ahead and tools for moving forward, but that's not all. You can see a way of thinking with joy about the world and a heartfelt understanding of being thankful for what comes next. Embrace the journey. Changing the way that you think about being well is a giant step in the right direction.

Sometimes when the two of us sit together and daydream, our thoughts wander to the future. Kat sees quieter days, sipping tea on a porch, watching the world go by, traveling to new places, and quiet time in the mountains. Nancy sees the chance to catch up on her reading and to spend some time at a cottage near the beach.

As we talk together about the future, we can also picture ourselves with more physical challenges. We may one day need help with walking, or maybe we will no longer be able to drive. Kat may require creative adaptive devices to help her use her hands. Nancy may need help going up stairs. Neither of us relishes the idea of losing function, but we no longer fear and dread it either. By daydreaming about how we will navigate challenges, we accept the possibility and integrate it into our own experiences.

When the day comes that we need assistance with movement, we have talked—and laughed—about having the finest, most decorated items around. As she has shared, Kat loves color and she loves polka dots, and we both like to make a little splash. If we need a walker, scooter, or wheelchair one day, it will be a colorful, well-adorned, one-of-a-kind device. Kat will have a flag, cozy quilted pillows, or hand grips, attached fabric bags to carry with her the things that bring her joy—maybe a small watercolor palette and sketchbook to record the day's events or the fresh bloom from a rose bush. Nancy will carry a pair of well-loved binoculars and call out the names of exotic birds that she imagines we might see along the way. Why look, it's a blue-throated hillstar.

Kat can also picture a lovely upright three wheeled bicycle with a big basket, and maybe an umbrella for the damp days (we get many of these in the Pacific Northwest). She will, for sure, have a delicate-sounding bell that gently alerts others to her presence. She thinks she will choose a vintage sort and hang it on a lovely velvet ribbon.

You see, the practice of finding joy allows us to find it no matter what the day might bring. We don't dread the days ahead, partly because we try hard to keep our focus on the present, but also because we believe that the practice of being well today will carry with us being well tomorrow and all the days that follow. It is simply our way of being now.

Here's one more thing before we go. We have introduced some of our friends in the previous pages, and hopefully you enjoyed reading about Jeff, Karen, Marilyn, Kerry Rae, and the others. We are thinking ahead to the friends we have yet to meet—people who have read this far, like you.

We look forward to meeting you on the journey one day soon and hearing *your* story.

❋ AFTERWORD

We worked for three years to make our dream of attending the World Parkinson Congress in Japan happen. One day, when we were reading about Kyoto, a photograph of bright reddish gates—called torii—at the Fushimi Inari shrine caught our attention. The gates seemed to shimmer, catching the sunlight, and rippling as if they were fabric instead of wood.

Like doorways, the torii gates are said to mark the transition from the mundane to the revered. During our planning stages, it became clear to us that we wanted to visit the shrine that had so inspired us. Seeing the torii was to become one of the high points of our trip to Japan.

Even though we arrived at the shrine early in the day, we were far from the only ones who were walking up the first steps. There were hundreds and hundreds of people already there. We started climbing in lockstep with the crowd. There were young and old visitors, families, individuals, observant Buddhists, and irreverent Americans. The cacophony of many languages found our ears. Occasionally someone posed for a photograph and the whole procession would stop and wait for them.

We had read in a travel book that the shrine had 10,000 torii gates, and that number had seemed manageable to us. Imagine our surprise when we learned that there are over 32,000 torii gates and over 50 flights of stairs. As you continue further, even when it appears that you have reached the top of the stairs, there are more to climb.

The lessons that we learned from climbing all the unexpected stairs at the shrine were similar to all that we have learned about Parkinson's.

The more we come to understand, through research and study, the more possibilities we have to reduce symptoms or discover a new medicine or—knock on wood, find a cure—and still there are new complications and surprises.

It took us more than two hours to reach the top of the shrine. By then, the crowd had moved on for the day, leaving hardly anyone except us—two women with Parkinson's disease. We knew the steep path still held surprises and would likely tap all our energy. So, we did what people do every day: we put one foot forward, and then the next. Slowly and steadily, we climbed. And we were amazed and thankful to be able to do so.

✳ ACKNOWLEDGEMENTS

Thank you to Eve Goodman, for her help and encouragement. Eve gave us more than just her time. Her belief in this book kept us going. She is a true professional and friend.

Thank you to Kimberly Berg and the Rebel Fit fighters, for early-morning workouts and non-stop encouragement. Coach Kimberly is a rock star, and she is "brave, mighty, sexy, and strong."

Thank you to Kerry Rae Connolly, for reading early editions, being our sounding board and cheering us on every step of the way.

Thank you to Karen Meadows, for her unwavering support and mentorship. We learned so much from you.

Thank you to Leslie Tuomi, for her encouragement, boundless energy and fantastic style, week after week.

Thank you to Elephants Deli for fueling us with caffeine and giving us a place to write and talk, and to say hello to the players at the morning cribbage table.

To Harry Bondareff, thank you for helping us to remember that life is precious. May you be finding all that is beauty and grace on the other side.

✳ FURTHER READING

We have read and written about a lot of books and listened to a lot of podcasts while we were preparing this work. Here are some of our favorites.

The Book of Joy: Lasting Happiness in a Changing World, Dalai Lama, Reverend Desmond Tutu and Douglas Carlton.

Ending Parkinson's Disease: A Prescription for Action, Ray Dorsey, Todd Sherer, Michael Okun, and Bastiaan Bloem.

Every Victory Counts Manual, Davis Phinney Foundation.

Hardwiring Happiness, Rick Hansen.

How to Live Well with Chronic Pain and Illness: A Mindful Guide, Toni Bernhard.

Searching for Normal: The Story of a Girl Gone Too Soon, Karen Meadows.

The Second Mountain: The Quest for a Moral Life, David Brooks.

Welcome to the YOPD Club: 10 Inspirational Stories From 10 People Living With Young Onset Parkinson's Disease, Christian Hageseth and William J Braddock.

✳ RESOURCES

WORLD PARKINSON COALITION
www.worldparkinsoncoalition.org

A non-religious, non-political, and non-profit organization concerned with the health and welfare of people living with Parkinson's disease, their families, and caregivers. Host of World Parkinson Congress.

THE DAVIS PHINNEY FOUNDATION
www.davisphinneyfoundation.org

A non-profit with a mission to help people with Parkinson's live well with the disease. Founded by Davis Phinney, the former professional road bicycle racer and Olympic medal winner.

THE MICHAEL J FOX FOUNDATION
www.michaeljfox.org

The largest non-profit funder of Parkinson's disease research in the world. Dedicated to finding a cure for Parkinson's disease and ensuring the development of improved therapies for those living with Parkinson's today.

PARKINSON'S RESOURCES OF OREGON (PRO)
www.parkinsonsresources.org

A donor supported non-profit with the mission of advancing the quality of life for people with Parkinson's, their families, and caregivers. Three locations, hundreds of volunteers, and dedicated leadership.

PD AVENGERS

A global alliance of people with Parkinson's, their partners, and friends. Standing together to demand change in how the disease is seen and treated. Inspired by the book "Ending Parkinson's Disease." pdavengers.com

PD LEMONADE PODCAST WITH KAT HILL

A refreshing take on finding joy. Apple and Spotify podcasts.

SPOTLIGHT YOPD

A UK-based charity with a global reach, raising awareness of Young Onset Parkinson's Disease and providing support to those living with the condition, using resources both online and offline.

WHEN LIFE GIVES YOU PARKINSON'S PODCAST WITH LARRY GIFFORD

A first-hand account of what it is like to live with Parkinson's disease for Gifford, his family, and other members of the worldwide Parkinson's community. Apple podcasts.

✳ BIBLIOGRAPHY

Ahlskog, J Eric (2011). "Does vigorous exercise have a neuroprotective effect in Parkinson disease?" *Neurology* vol. 77,3 288-94.

Barry, Lynda (2014). Syllabus: Notes from an Accidental Professor. Drawn and Quarterly.

Bloem BR, Henderson EJ, Dorsey ER, Okun MS, Okubadejo N, Chan P, Andrejack J, Darweesh SKL, Munneke M. (2020). Integrated and patient-centred management of Parkinson's disease: a network model for reshaping chronic neurological care. *Lancet* Neurol. Jul;19(7):623-634. doi: 10.1016/S1474-4422(20)30064-8.

Bowlby, J. (1973). Separation. New York: Basic Books.

Braddock, William J. (2020). Welcome To The YOPD Club: 10 Inspirational Stories From 10 People Living With Young Onset Parkinson's Disease.

Buettner, Dan (2011) Thrive: Finding Happiness the Blue Zones Way. National Geographic.

Chan CL, Ng SM, Ho RT, Chow AY. (2006). "East meets West: applying Eastern spirituality in clinical practice." *J Clin Nurs.* Jul;15(7):822-32.

Chopra, Mallika (2015). Living With Intent, TEDx Talk San Diego https://www.tedxsandiego.com/transcripts/2015-talks/mallika-chopra/

Chopra, Mallika (2015). Living With Intent: My Somewhat Messy Journey to Purpose, Peace and Joy. Harmony Books, first ed.

Dahl, CJ; Wilson-Mendenhall, CD; Davidson, RJ (2020)."The plasticity of well-being: A training-based framework for the cultivation of human flourishing." *Proceedings of the National Academy of Sciences of the United States of America.* PMID 33288719 DOI: 10.1073/pnas.2014859117.

Da Silva, Franciele Cascaes et al. (2018). "Effects of physical exercise programs on cognitive function in Parkinson's disease patients: A systematic review of randomized controlled trials of the last 10 years." *PloS* one vol. 13,2 e0193113. 27 Feb. 2018.

Dalai Lama, Reverend Desmond Tutu and Douglas Carlton (2016) The Book of Joy: Lasting Happiness in a Changing World, Avery.

Dawson, T. (2021). The Genetic Link to Parkinson's Disease. Retrieved 8/27/2021. https://www.hopkinsmedicine.org/health/conditions-and-diseases/parkinsons-disease/the-genetic-link-to-parkinsons-disease

Dölen G, Darvishzadeh A, Huang KW, Malenka RC. (2013). Social reward requires coordinated activity of nucleus accumbens oxytocin and serotonin. *Nature.* Sep 12;501(7466):179-84.

Dorsey, R., Sherer, T., Okun, M., Bloem, B. (2020) "Ending Parkinson's Disease: A Prescription for Action," *PublicAffairs.*

Dupre ME, Nelson A. (2016) Marital history and survival after a heart attack. *Soc Sci Med.* Dec;170:114-123

Filkowski, M; Cochran, RN; Haas, Brian (2016). Altruistic behavior: mapping responses in the brain. *Neurosci Neuroecon.* 5: 65-75. DOI: 10.2147/NAN.S87718. Accessed 7/19/2021.

Flanagan, R. (2021). Women with Parkinson's Disease: the effect of female hormones on Parkinson's symptoms. April 14. Cure Parkinson's Trust webinar "Women and Parkinson's disease: the hormonal impact " April 26. PMD Alliance webinar " Women's Hormones and Parkinson's Disease."

Garland, Eric L., Fredrickson, Barbara Ann, Kring, M., Johnson, David P., Meyer, Piper S., Penn, David L. (2010) *Clinical Psychology Review*, Volume 30, Issue 7, November, Pages 849-864. "Upward spirals of positive emotions counter downward spirals of negativity: Insights from the broaden-and-build theory and affective neuroscience on the treatment of emotion dysfunctions and deficits in psychopathology."

Gawande, Atul (2014). Being Mortal: Medicine and What Matters in the End. Metropolitan Books.

Giroux, Monique and Farris, Sierra (2019). Every Victory Counts: Essential Information and Inspiration for a Lifetime of Wellness with Parkinson's Disease, fifth ed. Davis Phinney Foundation For Parkinson's.

Gjerstad, M D et al. (2007). "Insomnia in Parkinson's disease: frequency and progression over time." *Journal of Neurology, Neurosurgery, and Psychiatry* vol. 78,5 (2007): 476-9.

Holmes, T. & Rahe, R. (1967). "The Social Readjustment Rating Scale." *Journal of Psychosomatic Research,* 11(2), 213–218. https://doi.org/10.1016/0022-3999(67)90010-4.

Holt-Lunstad, PhD, Julianne. (2017). "The Potential Public Health Relevance of Social Isolation and Loneliness: Prevalence, Epidemiology, and Risk Factors." *Public Policy & Aging Report*, Vol 27, Issue 4, 127–130, https://doi.org/10.1093/ppar/prx030.

Inzelberg R. (2013). "The awakening of artistic creativity and Parkinson's disease." *Behav Neurosci.* Apr;127(2):256-61.

Isaacs, Tom (2015). "The road to fulfilment from diagnosis to advocacy," *Parkinson's Life*. https://parkinsonslife.eu/the-road-to-fulfilment-from-diagnosis-to-advocacy/

Johansson H, Hagströmer M, Grooten WJA, Franzén E. (2020). Exercise-Induced Neuroplasticity in Parkinson's Disease: A Metasynthesis of the Literature. *Neural Plast.* 2020 Mar 5;2020:8961493.

Johns Hopkins Medicine (2021) August 10. "How Parkinson's Disease Is Diagnosed." Hopkins Medicine. https://www.hopkinsmedicine.org/health/treatment-tests-and-therapies/how-parkinson-disease-is-diagnosed.

Kay DB, Tanner JJ, Bowers D. (2018) "Sleep disturbances and depression severity in patients with Parkinson's disease." *Brain Behav.* Jun;8(6).

Kessler, S. (1989). "Psychological aspects of genetic counseling: VI. A critical review of the literature dealing with education and reproduction." *American Journal of Medical Genetics.* First published: November, https://doi.org/10.1002/ajmg.1320340310.

Kim, Eric S. and Konrath, Sara H (2016). "Volunteering is prospectively associated with health care use among older adults". *Social Science & Medicine*, Volume 149, January, Pages 122-129.

Kim, Linda, et al (2019). "What makes team communication effective: a qualitative analysis of interprofessional primary care team members' perspectives." *Journal of Interprofessional Care.* Nov/Dec2019, Vol. 33 Issue 6, p836-838. 3p.

Kois, Dan (2011). Lynda Barry Will Make You Believe In Yourself. *New York Times* magazine, Oct. 27, 2011.

Kroenke, C.H., Michael, T.L., Poole, E.M., Kwan, M.L., Nechuta, S., Leas, E., Caan, B.J., Pierce, J., Shu, X., Zheng, Y., Chen, W.Y. (2016). Postdiagnosis social networks and breast cancer mortality in the After Breast Cancer Pooling Project, *Cancer,*

Kubler—Ross, Elisabeth and Kessler, David (2007) On Grief and Grieving: Finding the Meaning of Grief Through the Five Stages of Loss, Scribner.

Lawton, R.N., Gramatki, I., Watt, W. et al. (2021). "Does Volunteering Make Us Happier, or Are Happier People More Likely to Volunteer? Addressing the Problem of Reverse Causality When Estimating the Wellbeing Impacts of Volunteering." *J Happiness Stud* 22, 599–624. https://doi.org/10.1007/s10902-020-00242-8.

Lewin Group (2019). Economic Burden and Future Impact of Parkinson's Disease, Final report. July 5. Report supported by the Michael J Fox Foundation. https://www.michaeljfox.org/sites/default/files/media/document/2019 Parkinson's Economic Burden Study—FINAL.pdf.

Lewis C, Annett L, Davenport S, Hall A, Lovatt P. (2016). Mood changes following social dance sessions in people with Parkinson's disease. *Journal of Health Psychology*; 21(4): 483–492.

Lidstone, SC (2014). "Great expectations: the placebo effect in Parkinson's disease." *Handbook Exp Pharmacology*;225:139-47.

Metcalfe-Roach, A, Yu, A.C., Golz, E., Cirstea, M., Sundvick, K., Kilger, D., Foulger, L.H., Mackenzie, M., Finlay, B.B., Appel-Cresswell, S. (2021). MIND and Mediterranean Diets Associated with Later Onset of Parkinson's Disease. *Movement Disorders*, Vol 36, No 4, p 977-984.

Mjåset, Christer (2018). TEDx Oslo. "4 questions you should always ask your doctor." https://www.ted.com/talks/christer_mjaset_4_questions_you_should_always_ask_your_doctor

National Institute on Aging (2017). "Parkinson's Disease." Retrieved 8/27/2021. https://www.nia.nih.gov/health/parkinsons-disease.

PD Avengers (2020). PD Avengers Origin Story: How a global alliance of advocates united with a common goal of ending Parkinson's, https://www.pdavengers.com/originstory.com/origin-story, www.pdavengers.com

Pew Research Center (2013). Pew Research Center Social & Demographic Trends. "Emotional Ties." https://www.pewsocialtrends.org/2013/01/30/emotional-ties/

Pinker, Susan (2017). TED Talk, "The Secret to Living Longer May Be Your Social Life." https://www.ted.com/talks/susan_pinker_the_secret_to_living_longer_may_be_your_social_life/transcript

Quaid, K. 1992 (published in 1994). "Streamlining genetic counseling for broader application." In Fullarton, J. (ed.) *Proceedings of the Committee on Assessing Genetic Risks*. Washington, D.C.: National Academy Press.

Rimon A, Shalom S, Wolyniez I, Gruber A, Schachter-Davidov A, Glatstein M. (2016). "Medical Clowns and Cortisol levels in Children Undergoing Venipuncture in the Emergency Department: A Pilot Study." *Isr Med Assoc J.* Nov;18(11):680-683.

Roberts, Kelly Rae (2021) www.kellyraeroberts.com.

Samson, Kurt (2011) "Stronger Social Support Shown to Improve Early Breast Cancer Outcomes." *Oncology Times*: October 10, 2011—Volume 33—Issue 19—p 36-38.

Schrag A, Hovris A, Morley D, Quinn N, Jahanshahi M. "Young- versus older-onset Parkinson's disease: impact of disease and psychosocial consequences." *Mov Disord.* 2003 Nov;18(11):1250-6. doi: 10.1002/mds.10527. PMID: 14639664.

Seidl, Santiago and Potashkin (2014). "The emerging role of nutrition in Parkinson's disease." *Front Aging Neuroscience*, March 7.

Sowislo, J.F. & Orth, U. (2013). "Does low self-esteem predict depression and anxiety? A meta-analysis of longitudinal studies." *Psychological Bulletin* 139(1) 213-240.

Stuckey, Heather L and Nobel, Jeremy (2019). "The Connection Between Art, Healing and Public Health: A Review of the Current Literature." *The Journal of Public Health.*

Vandenberg, et al. (2019). "Mindfulness-based lifestyle programs for the self-management of Parkinson's disease in Australia." *Health Promotion International*, Vol. 34 Issue 4, p668-676. 9p.

Wexler, N. (1992). "The Tiresias complex: Huntington's disease as a paradigm of testing for late-onset disorders." *FASEB Journal* 6:2820-2825.

Wikipedia (2021) Definition of Joy, January 2021.

✳ ABOUT THE AUTHORS

Kat Hill is a retired Nurse Midwife who delivered over 800 babies in her career. She retired after being diagnosed with young onset Parkinson's disease in 2015. Now she writes, speaks, and advocates for living with resilience. She also hosts a podcast called PD Lemonade that you can find on iTunes and Spotify. Kat and her husband Ken 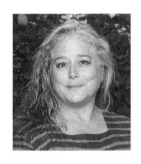 have raised three bright and spirited children in Portland, Oregon. When not traveling with her husband, she can be found painting, recording, or sewing with Baxter, her Yorkshire Terrier, by her side.

Nancy Peate grew up in Colorado. After working as a software technical writer, she returned to the classroom to get a master's degree in Library Science and worked until recently retiring as an adult reference librarian. Nancy has lived with Parkinson's disease since 2014. She's found a supportive community and participates in sev- 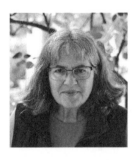 eral activities for people living with Parkinson's, including non-contact boxing classes, a dance troupe, and a drumming circle. Nancy and her husband, Rob, have a son in college. They live in Portland, Oregon.

Shortly after Nancy was diagnosed, through serendipity and good fortune, she met her friend, speaking partner, and co-author Kat Hill. Together, Nancy and Kat speak to community groups and conferences around the world about learning how to thrive after a diagnosis of chronic illness. This is their first book.